A Cultural Biography of the Prostate

A Cultural Biography
of the Prostate

Ericka Johnson

The MIT Press

Cambridge, Massachusetts | London, England

The MIT Press would like to thank the anonymous peer reviewers who provided comments on drafts of this book. The generous work of academic experts is essential for establishing the authority and quality of our publications. We acknowledge with gratitude the contributions of these otherwise uncredited readers.

This book was set in Stone Serif and Stone Sans by Jen Jackowitz. Printed and bound in the United States of America.

Library of Congress Cataloging-in-Publication Data

Names: Johnson, Ericka, 1973- author.
Title: A cultural biography of the prostate / Ericka Johnson, The MIT Press.
Description: Cambridge, Massachusetts : The MIT Press, [2021] | Includes bibliographical references and index.
Identifiers: LCCN 2020050487 | ISBN 9780262543040 (paperback)
Subjects: LCSH: Prostate--Popular works.
Classification: LCC RC899 .J64 2021 | DDC 616.6/5--dc23
LC record available at https://lccn.loc.gov/2020050487

10 9 8 7 6 5 4 3 2 1

To Dad

Contents

The stars we are given. The constellations we make.

Rebecca Solnit[1]

Introduction

It's the third time since midnight. Your feet slide off the bed. There is a draft on the floor. Cold air tenses the muscles in your shoulders as you shift into a sitting position. You reluctantly leave the warm bed and stand up.

The body next to you grumbles at being disturbed again and turns toward the wall. You walk to the bathroom and stand at the toilet. And stand there. And stand there. And finally, a small stream escapes. A pause. A few more drips. You don't flush, just to spare your partner the extra noise. Crawl back into bed. Try to push the worry about what is wrong out of your head, wolf-hour fears of cancer, expanding middle lobes, and peeing like an old man . . . about being an old man. . . . And you try to go back to sleep. Perhaps this has become your nightly routine.

Or, maybe you have gradually realized that you know where the bathroom is at each café, grocery store, and shopping center in a ten-mile radius. You have noticed that you are stopping at the gas station to take a bathroom break more and more frequently. Long car rides become trying, and events like movies, plays, or concerts are interrupted—possibly even avoided—because of the need to pee in the middle of them.

Or, maybe there are changes in your sex life that make you think there might be something wrong. Perhaps you are worried that if something is wrong, treating it is going to radically alter the intimacy you and your partner share.

Whatever the cause, I suspect that if you are reading this book, you are probably worried about the prostate.

You are not alone. Sometimes, I think that we are *all* worried about the prostate. Men are worried about their own prostates, and probably the prostates of those close to them. Women are worried about the prostates of the men they love, be those husbands or partners, fathers or sons. Even young people are worried about their fathers' and grandfathers' prostates—and sometimes their own. This is partly because we, as a population, are getting older, and ageing has traditionally been associated with prostate problems. There are more older prostates to worry about. And in the last decade there has been an increased awareness about prostate cancer, a big source of prostate angst. Prostates are the topic of TV shows, podcasts, and pharmaceutical commercials. Newspapers write about them. Doctors ask about them. Everyone is talking about them—often in hushed and serious tones. No wonder we are worried.

And it isn't just the general public that is concerned about the prostate. The medical community is, too.

For the last fifteen years, I've been researching men's health from within medical sociology, and I assure you that the prostate has appeared in a lot of the medical information that I have been studying.[2] When I first noticed this, I began to wonder where, when, and how it started to be a problem. I wanted to know why the prostate always seemed to be lurking on the periphery of many men's health issues. But what really triggered the research this book is based on was the explanatory comment I found over and over in various medical columns and websites, when a patient would present with diffuse pain and urination problems. The diagnosis: "It is probably the prostate that is haunting him."[3] This suggestion seemed in line with the general understanding of the prostate as a man's constant torment.[4] These two descriptions and their implicit ambiguity reflect a good deal of the prostate "knowledge" that I have encountered in my research journey. And it is a perfect example of the undeniably interesting element of medical knowledge about the prostate: it is a gland that haunts. What could be more interesting than a gland that haunts? And what on earth could that description of the prostate be doing in medical diagnostic practice?

A Cultural Biography

That the prostate could be a gland that haunts is, of course, only a metaphor or a trope. The prostate is, still, just a gland located directly under the bladder. And yet it is so much more. Our understandings of the body—how we imagine various parts of them, what we think those parts do, what problems they are blamed for—are intimately related to the metaphors, tropes, and narratives we tell about them or use to describe or contextualize them.[5] How we and medical professionals describe the prostate, and the words it is embedded in, both reveal and impact on what we think it is, what we think it does, and what we think we should do to or about it. In this book I will discuss what understandings of the prostate are influenced by (and reveal about) tropes of masculinity, sexuality, ageing, and health, both in historical material and in current medical texts and practices. Therefore, I hope it will interest students of urology, medical practitioners, public health officials, and other people concerned about prostate health. But because I present results from an interdisciplinary approach to studying the body that employs ideas and concerns from the medical humanities, I also hope the book will be interesting to those working in that field, in particular medical sociologists and historians of medicine.

I am writing a biography of the prostate. In the same way as biographies use varied and different memories and archival sources to tell the story of a person, I will be using varied and different sources to tell many stories of the prostate. In a traditional biography, it is legitimate to employ a mix of sources like written documents, official information, personal memories, and interviews. Biography as a literary genre can show that different contacts—professionals, relatives, friends, lovers—have different understandings of a person and, in the best of cases, a biography tries to create a rich and detailed narrative about the complexity of a person's life.

This approach can work for objects, too. Even glands. I write about heterogeneous aspects, conflicting understandings, and culturally contextual contours of the prostate, and the way its diverse and multifeatured identity reflects the changing cultural and historical aspects of the bodies it is in.[6] I draw inspiration from medical sociology, science and technology studies, feminist theory, and, in particular, new materialities,[7] teasing apart what we think the prostate is and what we use the prostate to think about. I am also inspired by the way the concept of *cultural biographies* of objects within anthropology was used to articulate the tenuousness of meaning and identity as objects are classified and reclassified, as they change context and are experienced.[8] Biographies often present conflicting ideas about their subject; one truth and one dominant narrative can hold for a while and then be replaced. Or there can be two different images of a person—a private and a public, for example—that coexist at the same time. And opinion about a person (or object) can change over time. A cultural-biographical approach lets me discuss the multiple and temporal narratives about the prostate, its different appearances and characteristics in different discourses, how different people think of it in different ways. The trope of biography will also allow me to spend some time writing about how the prostate becomes a significant object of meaning-making in the lives of men for whom it is a problem.[9] It is not only the prostate that has a biography; the prostate plays a significant role in the biographies of those for whom it is troublesome.

The prostate exists—it is a thing—but it is also a scientific object of study, an object that medicine explores and treats. Scientific objects, as Daston points out, have a history. They become entangled in "webs of cultural significance, material practices, and theoretical derivations."[10] Using the word entangled—and I will use it quite a lot—is a way of reminding myself and the reader that the physical object, our ways of knowing about it, our ways of talking or writing, imaging or imagining it, are a messy, tangled node of relations. Tracing these relations means following the ways of knowing that are making the prostate more salient,[11] or producing it through material-discursive cuts.[12] Or creating a constellation out of the stars.[13] As I trace the production of constellations of meaning from the stars of a gland, I am going to be looking closely at the materialities of scientific practice that make prostate knowledge possible, the networks of human and nonhuman actors which accompany it.[14] Through observations from ethnographic research and interviews, analysis of historical material and current medical texts, I show how one can understand the prostate and its current ontological state through intersecting histories and actualities of medicine, the body, and gender. The book unveils the prostate gland, explaining what it is and what we know about it, but also—primarily—discusses how the prostate has discursively been connected to ageing, masculinity, sexuality, and health in the cultural *zeitgeist*. My argument is that those values, expectations, and norms about ageing, masculinity, sexuality, and health are entangled with the gland, which has consequences for the bodies seeking or offered medical treatment for the prostate.[15]

Much of the material I have found employs cultural assumptions about hegemonic masculinities, heterosexuality, and "typical" male behavior in explaining the prostate, and much of my analysis teases out and articulates how culturally specific concepts of male, man, heterosexual, and masculine are engaged and employed in connection with the prostate. This is, of course, not to say that all bodies with a prostate identify with those understandings of male and masculine, or that all bodies with a prostate are cis male.[16] You may have noticed that I used the terms men and women in the narrative at the beginning of this introduction, and I will largely continue with these glosses throughout the book, reflecting the way binary sex is present in the majority (*vast* majority) of medical literature about the prostate—and how this paradigm dominates the systems of specialist care that bodies with prostates encounter, something that becomes poignantly relevant in the discussion in chapter 4 about prostatitis. By using this gloss, men and women, I am not saying it is the only or the correct way to talk about bodies with prostates. However, when talking about prostate cancer, prostatitis, and other prostate problems causing frequent or difficult urination, it is the cis man's prostate and the socially male body which most people are referring to, and which appears in many of the social aspects related to the prostate's cultural contours that are going to be examined here. Those concepts (and related values, expectations, and norms about heteronormative, cis male masculinity) impact on care options for those who identify as heterosexual and those who don't, and those who are cis male and those who are not.

Interdisciplinary Research Methods

The medical humanities constitute a rapidly growing field—sort of soft at the edges—that engages with and incorporates theoretical and methodological ideas and tools from across the humanities and social sciences. From this field, I draw inspiration in examining the metaphors and tropes used to describe the body and its pathologies, as mentioned above, along with a critical stance toward the institution of medicine[17] and its various incarnations in different times and places.[18] A prominent element of the "critical" stance in the medical humanities is a willingness to engage different fields of science and different ways of doing research: to take an interdisciplinary approach.[19]

This book does that. It grew from a research project I led which involved nine researchers working collaboratively across anthropology, medical sociology, history of medicine, STS and medicine, sexual therapy, and feminist technoscience studies. We all approached the ageing prostate as an evocative object, but from our different starting points. We looked at and saw different things as we traced the contours and textures of discourses that define and describe the prostate in different times and places. Some of us examined cultural and historical constructions of the prostate as a node of pain, discomfort, and angst, using interviews and archive material. Others explored the medical discourses (including what we call material-semiotic practices, or the way things and ideas together produce meaning) which enact the prostate as a discrete anatomical object to be tested through blood samples, physically examined in the body, and surgically removed. We variously used ethnographic observation, interviews with professionals, and analysis of medical articles and guidelines. And as some of the subprojects delineated how the prostate is known and invoked in the body and in its absence, after surgical removal, we also employed discourse analysis of written and interview material with men who have or have had prostates. We predominantly relied on qualitative methods. As I have written up my research results from this study, I have used material from interviews that I conducted, discourse analysis of medical literature and cultural imaginaries that I collected, and theoretical insights I gained in conversations with urologists and other medical sociologists. But I am also drawing on results from each of the projects my colleagues conducted and the conversations we have had throughout the study (referenced and cited—you will meet their work throughout the following chapters). In this way, I hope to weave our conclusions together to present a rich image of the prostate as a cultural phenomenon.

There are particular methodological challenges and benefits of doing interdisciplinary work like this. Our research team included social scientists and humanities researchers, but also a sexologist, and we all had very different understandings of what knowledge is and our role in making it. During our shared conversations, we needed to talk openly about what it meant to work with empirical data from interviews, observations, and archive materials, because not all of us had the same ideas. I had expected some of these conversations to become a bit awkward, and figured it would probably be most difficult when we were coauthoring with the sexologist—who worked at a urology department and could have been expected to be much more prone to positivist knowledge paradigms than, say, those of us in gender studies. But it was actually the most difficult (in a fun, challenging way, I have to add—we really did all get along almost all of the time) when we were collaborating between and amongst ourselves, as social scientists and humanities researchers. For example, the PhD candidate, (now Dr.) Björk, had a historian as one supervisor, and me—a professor of gender and society—as another. In many ways, this student was the one who actually did "interdisciplinary work" in her attempt to write a dissertation that could be approved by a committee of historians, but also integrated a new materialities-inspired analysis of her data. It worked, thanks to her efforts and diplomacy, and maybe this sort of uncomfortable parenting is the most productive way to do interdisciplinarity. I'm not sure how much the rest of us in the group did interdisciplinary work—mostly we worked separately, then had interdisciplinary conversations during our meetings and seminars. Some of these conversations appeared, later, in our analytical work, but not always, and not usually that influentially.

I think this can be seen clearly in the anthology we produced as a collective.[20] We each wrote a chapter, and we worked through these chapters together during a series of workshops. This meant that we were able to refer to the work of the other authors in our own chapters, and to come to some general statements together in its introduction (thanks largely to the efforts of the editor, Dr. Björkman), but we didn't have to integrate each other's theoretical or epistemological approaches into our own writing. A more integrative interdisciplinarity is much more difficult. An anthology is a gentle, forgiving place to publish interdisciplinary conversations—while publishing, on the other hand, is one of those aspects of interdisciplinary work that can be difficult. How does one find journals interested in such studies? How can one convince the top journals in one's field to step beyond the traditional disciplinary boundaries (methodological approaches, theoretical conversations) to accept interdisciplinary work? Or how to convince one's disciplinary peers to value publications that appear in (often newer, less well known) journals which accept interdisciplinary contributions, especially during all-important career steps like tenure, and funding applications? Having grown up academically in the field of science and technology studies, during a period when it was consolidating into a field after starting as a new, interdisciplinary area, I tend to think that these problems solve themselves with time. But that is neither an easy nor a generous thing to say to younger colleagues who are dealing with all those moments in the early career, moments which require convincing older peers that one is both pushing the envelope and squarely contributing to one's own discipline.

The institutional framework within which a project like this can be run is also important, and I had the great good fortune to be at a department built on interdisciplinarity as a concept. My departmental head did not bat an eyelid when I came to him and said I wanted to hire two sociologists, two anthropologists, a historian, a gender studies researcher, an undefined graduate student, and a sexologist—who was going to be employed at a hospital, no less, and needed money to be sent there. I recognize the luxury of being able to do this without (too much) administrative trouble (thank you, Linköping University!). It allowed me to gather the group in relatively close quarters, and facilitated prostate-project lunches, coffee conversations, joint seminar presentations, and even the integration of our research into undergraduate and graduate teaching.

Working together in the same corridors and meeting each other in the lunch room, classrooms, and seminar rooms also meant that we had to develop an understanding for what the other team members thought were legitimate ways to do research. What is data? What can one do with it? Why does one have theory, and to what end does one use it in an analysis? We learned to probe gently when one of us (usually the historian) reacted in surprise to another person's use of (often archive) material. We found ourselves having shared conversations about the importance of context—both from a historian's point of view, and from one inspired by feminist technoscience and Haraway's insistence on the contingency of knowledge production.[21] And we tried to make sure that we were clear in how we used ethnographic observations, interview material, and discursive analysis of texts, so that we could be respectful of context and contingency (in historical and present-day studies) rather than making it appear as if we were cherry-picking the good stuff to support an argument (as our historian tended to suspect). And we all tried to work on using our material to open up further questions, rather than as facts for explaining how and why the world *is* in sweeping, generalizing, stabilizing terms. Instead, we tried to approach the minutiae of how the world (and, specifically, the prostate) is *becoming*.

These moments have been both challenging and enriching. We have had to ask why some of us are interested in the empirical material in completely different ways than others. How can, for example, irreverence for historical method be tamed? Should it be? Or how can historians engage with theory and question knowledge production practices in the archive material they access? Similarly, questions arose as the anthropology- and sociology-trained researchers engaged with urologists, nurses, psychologists, and sexologists, sometimes thinking along with them, other times using them as informants. We discussed what it meant to shift between those relational roles with one's colleagues/informants, ethically[22] and epistemologically, and what those shifts did with expectations of coauthorship, for example, or "impact," and how we wanted to intervene.[23]

These conversations and practices produced wrinkles in the research process, which we were generally able to iron out through open dialogue. But they also had implications for the knowledge we produced.

Why did I bother to do it this way? Why did I design this project to be interdisciplinary when I first applied for the grant? As I said, I'm working in the medical humanities and I "grew up" in science and technology studies. Interdisciplinarity has seeped into my marrow. I probably couldn't get rid of this approach if I tried. But I also believe it is very generative. By using the prostate as a case, and engaging a heterogeneous team of disciplinary researchers, I was able to get a better feel for the discursive, cultural contours of the prostate. But studying the prostate this way also demonstrates that a variety of different theoretical approaches to our medicalized bodies (and subjectivities) provide useful insights into how we understand ourselves, our anatomies, and our changing bodies as we age. And by being a bit promiscuous with theory and method, it was easy to address the different facets of the prostate as it appears in our cultural imaginary. How else could one integrate a discussion of the PSA test as a screening technology along with the historical understanding of a diseased prostate and a modern analysis of a diagnostic guideline? And then throw some sex and a gender analysis into the mix? One discipline and one theoretical approach would not have been enough to trace these contours the way I wanted to. Leading an interdisciplinary group let me draw from the insights different theoretical approaches can allow when analyzing the prostate, but also lifted the discussion to one of how we understand our anatomies and pathologies, in different times and different institutional frameworks.

Outline

These different times and institutional frameworks appear throughout the rest of the book, called forth by the various entanglements I set out to explore. In the first chapter, I start unraveling the "is" of the prostate, initially by discussing some of the biomedical understandings of it and some of the methods that exist for examining, imaging, and teaching about it. What the prostate does in our body is a big part of what it "is," but what tools and methods we have for knowing the prostate play a role in how well we can examine it and what sort of knowledge we can create about it. However, the way we talk about the prostate in general (and about prostate cancer in particular) also creates particular contours of the prostate today.

This discussion sets the stage for chapter 2, where I explore how the prostate came to be known, historically. After painting with broad brush-strokes a history of when it was "discovered" and how it came to be known as, specifically, a prostate, I spend some time looking at a period during the end of the 1800s when the prostate became the focus for surgical and medical interventions, but also became a tool for discussing appropriate masculinities and sexual behavior. Social values and norms appear to be intimately entangled with the prostate and its pathologies in the historical material, and these are teased out by the treatment options that were available at the time.

Chapter 3 returns to the present, and here I explore the diagnostic guidelines for benign prostate hyperplasia—when the prostate begins to grow again in older men. This is different from cancer—it is benign—but it can still cause serious problems with urination. Diagnosing this condition involves a series of tests that measure both urination practices and troubles, but also examination practices that try to say something about the prostate. Measurements of urination become indicators of an enlarged prostate, and thereby turn a practice (urinating) into a thing (the gland). As I unpack how this happens, though, I point out moments when social elements of life are bracketed into medical knowledge about the prostate, in ways not so dissimilar to the historical examples from the previous chapter.

Prostate problems are usually associated with the ageing male body. But in chapter 4, I discuss the diagnosis "prostatitis," a condition—or collection of symptoms—that is often applied to younger bodies with prostates. I follow the twists and turns of this disease and its treatments, tracing the institutional trajectories a body follows to end up with the diagnosis "prostatitis." Finally, I ask if those paths of binary gendered healthcare (we seek specialist care from urologists or gynecologists) are what produce the diagnosis, and consider what a nonbinary understanding of the body would do to the disease of prostatitis.

One cannot write about the prostate (today) without writing about prostate cancer, so in chapter 5, I bend to the forces of discourse and write about the PSA test, and in particular the debates about PSA screening. Using the case of Sweden—which has universal healthcare, but has decided not to offer PSA screening to the population—I trace the debate in medical literature and, interestingly, in other conversations as well, trying to nuance the understandings of expertise, health, and vulnerability that PSA screening awakens (and, sometimes, silences) in its path.

Finally, in chapter 6, I write about the incredible presence of the absent prostate—the way the prostate impacts on lives when it has been removed or destroyed in the name of health.

I ask that the reader keep in mind that this book is being written in Sweden and that much, but not all, of our research has been conducted here. We have relied on Swedish texts, but also work written in North America, the UK, and other parts of Europe, and some of our interviews have been conducted with men and healthcare professionals in other countries. There is a strong Northern European perspective that we bring to the conversation. But I would gently point out that the alleged international—from nowhere and for everywhere—evidence-based medicine perspective of the majority of texts we have read, and knowledge we have encountered, is also geographically and culturally located. The prostate and the prostate's diseases that are discussed here are entangled with concepts the body and the masculine subject also found in those locations and cultures. Which is, of course, the point. The prostate has cultural contours. The work presented here has tried to palpate some of them.

1
What Is the Prostate?

Early on in this study, I contacted the Stockholm Men's Sexual Health Clinic and asked to do some interviews with their staff. They have a fairly young clientele, and much of their care focuses on safe and healthy sexual practices. Because prostate problems usually occur in older men, I did not think they would have too many patients with prostate issues, but I felt I needed to do the interviews anyway, since a project about an issue so obviously related to men's health should have contact with a men's health clinic.

During an interview with one of the nurses working there, however, I realized that the prostate *was* very present in their clinical conversations. Even though this nurse's patients were mostly young men, he did not think it was at all odd that I wanted to speak about prostates. After first reminding me that the prostate is not only an organ that gets diseased, that it can also be an erotic zone, he said his main issue with the prostate was that most of his patients didn't know what it was, what it did, where it was located, or what could go wrong with it. Yet, still, many of them were extremely worried they might have prostate cancer. As soon as a young man had the slightest pain anywhere in the genital area, they came to him with a panicked concern about cancer. "We're talking twenty-year-olds," he said. "Twenty-year-olds don't get prostate cancer. And most of them don't even know *where* their prostate is. But all anyone ever talks about these days is prostate cancer. So everyone with an itch from a sexually transmitted infection is suddenly terrified they are going to die of cancer."

"Surely they know where the prostate is," I said, naively overestimating the amount of anatomical knowledge Swedish sex education provided. "Wouldn't they have learned that at school?"

"Nope," he said, shaking his head. "They don't know where it is or what it does. If I had one wish, it would be for a little film about the prostate. Something I could show to my patients that would explain the most basic facts about it and help me assure them that they do not have prostate cancer." Then he turned to his computer and brought up an example on YouTube, a short, animated movie that had gone viral a few years back, which compared sexual consent with accepting or declining a cup of tea.[1]

"This is what I want to have for the prostate. A film I can show my patients so we can then have a conversation about their anatomy."

"Oh." I looked back at him. "Perhaps we should make one."

I don't know why I said that. I don't make films. And I am not an anatomy expert. But as an academic, I am expected to collaborate with people outside the academy, and this seemed like an ideal way to do that, with people working in healthcare around questions related to the prostate. The nurse liked the idea, too. Together, he and I wrote a screenplay and hired some animators to make a short, informational film[2] about the prostate that could be shown in his clinic. We explained what the prostate is, where in the body it is found, what it does, that it can become infected, *and* that it is probably not developing cancer in a young man's body.

In principle, there is no new information in the film—anyone doing a thorough search on the Internet could find the same facts. We did try to avoid connecting the anatomical prostate with a socially male body, and we mentioned the association between the prostate and sexual pleasure, but neither of these stances is terribly radical or unusual at a men's sexual health clinic in Sweden. What I think is most interesting about the film, however, is that there was a need for it in the first place, a need which speaks both to the absence of the prostate in the standard sex education curriculum (in any case, in Sweden) and to the overt presence of the prostate (diseased with cancer) in the social imaginary. We are not educating our young adults about the prostate as an important anatomical component of the reproductive system, nor as a potential erotic zone, but we *are* bombarding them in the media with information about prostate cancer. No wonder all those young men were coming to the clinic afraid of their prostates—and afraid of cancer, impotence, and possibly death. That is what the prostate represents for many people today, and most people know very little else about it. This flickering of the prostate's presence/absence and the questions it triggers about when the prostate appears and when it disappears, as well as which types of prostates are present (diseased ones) and which are absent (healthy ones), points to the big question of what the prostate "is"; not just where in the body, but in our thoughts and worries. Tracing its cultural contours means unpacking what a prostate "is."

There are many parts of the body we tend not to know or think much about—the pancreas, for example, or the Skene's glands, or our appendix. These, like the prostate, function silently deep inside us until something goes wrong and they need to be treated or removed. And there are other parts of the body we think we have figured out, like the ovaries—credited with producing eggs and little else—but which, as we start to analyze what happens when they are removed, suddenly appear to be important parts of bigger systems affecting many other parts of our lives: sleep, memory, and mood.[3] The prostate is definitely one of these organs that we are only vaguely aware of when it is healthy. I remember one interview with a younger man—in his thirties—when he brought up the fact that he, too, had not really understood where the prostate was and what it did at the beginning of his experiences with prostate trouble. He embedded this reflection in a discussion of how well he knew the anatomy and function of the female body. ("I had always made a point of being very well informed about the female anatomy when I was younger. In fact, I was able to explain a thing or two about it to my girlfriend.") But, as he said, there had been nothing about the prostate in his human biology classes as a student, and he knew little about it before his urologist had pulled out a model and explained where it was. He had never really thought about the prostate . . . until it became a source of pain.

This is not necessarily all bad. Some philosophical theories of the body[4] remind us that the unknown, silent, invisible body is the healthy body—and that disease and pain trigger awareness of this body. We should, perhaps, be grateful that we do not know much about the prostate, and realize that it becomes apparent only when it is acting up. But, on the other hand, if the imaginary ghost of prostate cancer is going to be haunting men of all ages, it is probably a good thing for them to know a bit about what the prostate is.

So, what *is* the prostate?

As the rest of this book will demonstrate, "is" is a difficult word for critical social theorists, and I will be doing a lot of work to explore what a prostate "is" in different discourses by asking who is using the word, what are they trying to say with it, what is being said between the lines when talking about it, with the goal of clarifying what work the prostate as a concept is doing in different conversations. But if you were to meet that nurse I spoke with at the men's sexual health clinic, he would answer that question something like this (ideally, after showing you the film): The prostate is a collection of glands, blood vessels, and some muscles, and is enclosed in a membrane-like sheath of tissue. It is in the lower abdomen, not far from where the penis is attached to the body. It is about two inches above the little piece of skin between the testicles and the anus (called the perineum) and it rests on the muscles of the pelvic floor. It is hidden inside the body, which is why doctors have to put their finger in the man's rectum to examine it.

The prostate is located just under the bladder, and urine passes through it on its way out via the penis. It helps to produce ejaculate. It is related to the hormone system. In English and in Swedish, the prostate is found in bodies with a penis, almost always assumed to be cis men. It is often embedded in discourses associated with cultural aspects of masculinity, sexuality, and ageing. (OK, the nurse may not give you that last sentence, but it's relevant for the rest of the book.) In German there is a term for the female prostate, which is approximately homologous to the G-spot.[5] But usually the prostate is assigned to the male body, and often associated with age-related diseases.

If the prostate acts up, this tends to happen when a man gets older. We all know about prostate cancer. But it can also get infected and cause prostatitis. In addition, the prostate can start to grow again around the age of fifty. A healthy, adult prostate is about the size of a walnut. But, as it begins regrowth, in some older men it can get to be the size of a kiwi, or even a medium-sized lemon (and, on rare occasions, the size of a grapefruit).

The prostate is part of the endocrine system, and interacts with testosterone. What role hormones play in prostate diseases is still not completely clear, but hormones—especially testosterone—seem to be in the background somewhere. This is why some of the treatments for prostate problems involve hormone therapies—and some involve castration, as I will detail in chapter 2.

The prostate affects the ease and frequency with which a man urinates. When he goes to the bathroom, the urine leaves the bladder through a tube called the urethra. That tube goes out through the penis. But before it does, it also runs through the prostate. As one urologist told me, the prostate is a little bit like a ping pong ball with a cocktail straw through it. That "straw" starts in the bladder, and its other end exits through the penis. In between, the straw has to pass through the prostate. That same tube in the penis, the urethra, is used for the sperm to travel through when a man ejaculates. Sperm is made in the testicles, and two tubes take it from the testicles to the backside of the prostate. In the prostate it is mixed with other fluids (made in all of those little glands) and shot out from the prostate into the urethra, and then out through the penis. The smooth muscles in the prostate work together with other muscles in the pelvic floor to help the man ejaculate.

Since the same tube, the urethra, is used for both peeing and ejaculating, the prostate and muscle fibers in the bladder neck make sure that the sperm mixture does not go into the bladder by closing off the bladder during ejaculation. These structures also make sure that urine is not expelled during ejaculation. When a man *is* peeing, the prostate closes off the ejaculatory ducts, at least to a certain degree, to minimize the amount of urine that enters the prostate. One could say the prostate is a bit like a traffic cop, getting the right stuff into the urethra and out through the penis at the right time.

When a doctor talks about the prostate with a patient, it is possible that they will start talking about lobes or zones of the prostate. These are terms for the front and the back, the inside and the outside of the prostate, and are useful because different diseases originate from and affect different parts of the prostate. Cancer, for example, will often appear in the rear section of the prostate, which the doctor might call the peripheral zone or the posterior lobe. This can be felt during the rectal examination, when the doctor puts his or her finger in the man's anus. Benign prostate hyperplasia (BPH), on the other hand, usually affects the inside of the prostate, which is called the transitional zone, and makes urinating difficult by obstructing the urethra.[6]

These are things the prostate *does* when it is healthy or diseased. But what does a prostate look like? Unlike a pair of tonsils or a woman's cervix, it is not visible through any openings. And even though it can be felt through the wall of the anus, it cannot be seen by looking up it.

The technologies we have available to us for examining and imaging the body impact on what we see and how we represent it. Those available technologies impact on the knowledge produced about the body, be they the paraffin used to make blood vessels visible in a corpse prepared for dissection and anatomical sketching in the 1700s, or the visualization algorithms that process data produced by modern scanners.[7] This is particularly relevant for the prostate, because it is so hidden. Doctors need to use different technologies in order to visualize it, and what the prostate looks like depends on what technology is being used to make the images. Here are a few pictures of prostates, but taken with different types of visualization technologies (different high-tech cameras, so to speak). These technologies allow us to see aspects of the prostate, but for a lot of the diagnostic practices and the treatments used for prostate problems, it is not necessary to see the gland itself. Exceptions include when a doctor will use an ultrasound probe to estimate prostate size and to collect biopsy samples— this helps the doctor to see which part of the prostate they are collecting samples from—and when surgeons use laparoscopic technology during surgery, a technological development which has made prostate surgery much, much safer. An ultrasound image can also show if a prostate has shrunk after certain treatments.

Figure 1.1 shows a prostate during an ultrasound exam. Transrectal ultrasound was introduced into urology practice in the 1980s as a complement to biopsy practices, so urology clinics acquired, and urologists became familiar with, the technology. Since then it has also been added to the examination toolbox for enlarged prostates.[8] Ultrasound is thought to be particularly

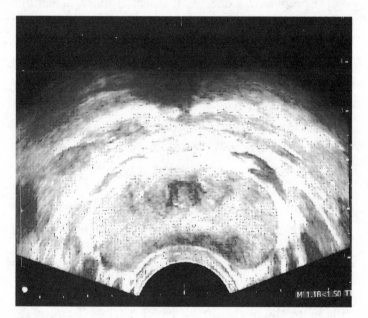

Figure 1.1
Image of a prostate taken by ultrasound, sourced by Carina Danemalm Jägervall.

useful for seeing the shape of the prostate, its different zones, and how it might be protruding into the bladder. The ultrasound examination creates an image of a man's prostate, and how it is shaped and positioned. In this picture, you can see a shadowy, gray, roundish area in the middle, which is the prostate. Don't worry if you don't really see a prostate in this picture. Keep in mind that ultrasound is rather like a black-and-white movie on the computer screen, not really a photograph. Remember all those ultrasound portraits you have seen of babies in the womb? And how hard it is to figure out what you are looking at before the expectant parents point out the feet and the head? The parents have been at the examination and watched the image being created on the screen as the ultrasound probe moves around the baby's body, so they know how the still, cross-cut image they are holding is related to the moving images of the baby. The same thing is true here. To make this picture, the doctor is moving the ultrasound handle around ever so slightly, and the image is being continuously refreshed on the screen. This makes it easier to see what is actually being shown, rather than trying to figure out what the prostate looks like from a still image like the one printed here. The prostate becomes visible through movements of the ultrasound apparatus, the professional conducting the exam, and the body.

Other ways of visualizing the prostate are with MRI or CT scans. The picture in figure 1.2 is from an MRI

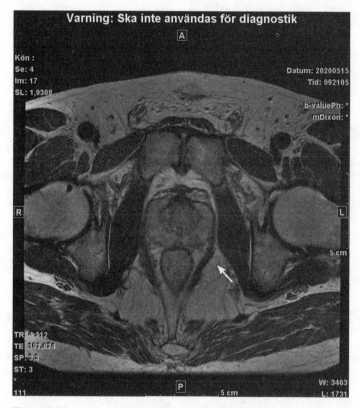

Figure 1.2
Image of a prostate taken by MRI, sourced by Carina Danemalm Jägervall.

scan. Both of these technologies produce a picture that is a cross-section of the body. In figure 1.2 you can see how the prostate is quite close to the rectum. You can see that by putting their finger in the rectum, the doctor could feel the backside of the prostate. This technology is now frequently used to look for signs of prostate cancer. Scanner technologies can also be used during cancer treatment to help localize and position radiation therapy. Because the prostate is very close to the bladder and the bowels, it can shift around a little bit as these are filled and emptied during the course of a day. Before shooting it with a radiation beam, radiation technicians want to make sure that the prostate is still in the same place they are aiming at, and they will often scan the body to check. If it has moved, they may ask the patient to wait a bit and try to have a bowel movement before they administer the radiation.

A more traditional way of showing what the prostate looks like is in anatomical drawings (figure 1.3). This is a painting that was done by an anatomy artist in 1943.[9] In it you clearly see how the urethra runs through the prostate from the bladder and out the penis. In its original color version, the prostate is tinted orange-beige, even though it is not really orange-beige inside the body. It *is* actually sort of pinkish, since there are lots of blood vessels in and around it, but there is no "standard" color for how prostates are depicted in anatomy drawings. What is standard is that color, shading, and lines are and have long been used to make distinctions between the different parts of the body, reproducing the edges of organs and glands as they were seen with dissection practices over the centuries, when drawing them for anatomy books and classes.

Photography also became used to illustrate books about prostate diseases and surgical methods as it

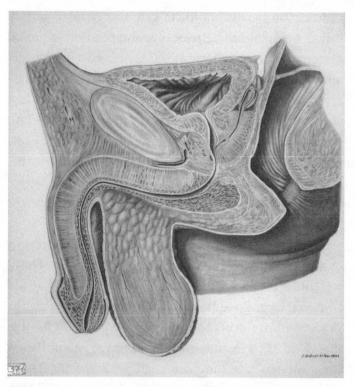

Figure 1.3
Anatomical drawing of the prostate. Lehrtafel Anatomisches Institut
der Universität Zürich, Zeichner: E. Brändli 30.09.1943. From the collection of the Archive of the History of Medicine, University of Zurich,
Signature IN 25 Nr. 417.

developed as a technology. One could take pictures of
what the removed prostate tissue looked like after an
operation. Figure 1.4 is an image from a book on prostatic surgery from 1906, showing a prostate outside
the body and separate from the surrounding tissues or

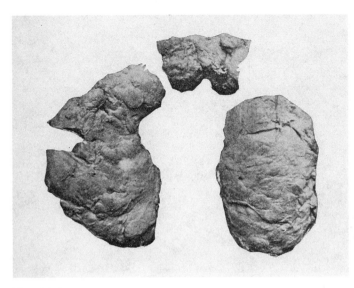

Figure 1.4
Photograph in H. Young, *Studies on Hypertrophy and Cancer of the Prostate*, Johns Hopkins Hospital Reports Vol. XIV (Baltimore: Johns Hopkins University Press, 1906), 35.

anatomical structures. Here the prostate becomes even more distinctly a discrete organ rather than a part of the genital system. And it became this because it had been identified as diseased, and removed.

Compare that to this picture of the prostate, a screen shot from the computer monitor on a robotic surgical instrument used to remove prostates, today (figure 1.5). When I first saw this picture, I had to have the doctor explain to me what was the prostate and what was surrounding tissue, because it was not immediately obvious, at least not from the visual image. When surgeons

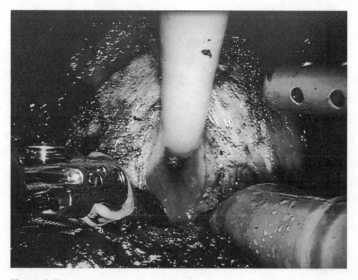

Figure 1.5
Image of a prostate taken during laparoscopic surgery, sourced by Carina Danemalm Jägervall.

are using these robotic instruments, the picture on the screen is magnified, to help them see the minute details of what they are cutting and cauterizing. This helps the surgeons to see the prostate a little better. But to determine which tissues are what, they also rely on how the different tissues respond to their instruments as they manipulate them, how they stretch or move, how the light reflects off them. The real body is not as easy to interpret as a still-life anatomy drawing with labeled parts, but it gives clues as it is poked and prodded, cut and cauterized.

The anatomy poster in figure 1.3 comes from the collection at the Medical History Museum and Library, University of Zurich, Switzerland.[10] When I was there doing some historical research, one of the archivists also showed me wax figures from their collection. We were down in the "basement" of the library, several floors underground, in what was a large, basketball-court-sized vault carved out of the Swiss Alps. In it were row after row of steel shelving that held medical paraphernalia from throughout the ages, pictures and models of parts of the body, glass jars with old body parts, skeletons, teeth, skulls. . . . I had asked if they had anything in their collection that dealt with the prostate, either images portraying it or instruments to measure or treat it. The archivist found this (figure 1.6)[11] on one of the upper shelves: the prostate in wax, modeled along with the rest of the male genitalia. It is a framed relief. On it, the different parts of the body are not labeled, which is what made her suspect that it had been produced to sell to European medical doctors who would have hung it on their office walls. Reliefs like this would have been a decoration meant to show off the doctor's knowledge. It, and several others in the series that they had there, were undated. But, on the basis of the old newspaper on the back of one of the frames, on what is known about the history of wax modeling in Switzerland, and on the medical pictures they seem to be copied from, the archivist suspected they had been made in the late

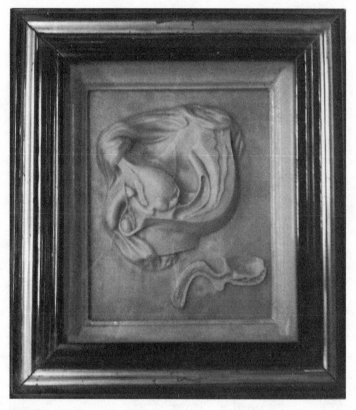

Figure 1.6
Wax model of the prostate. Probably Josef Benedikt Curiger (1754–1819) from Einsiedeln. From the Medical Collection, Institute of Evolutionary Medicine, University of Zurich, Inv. Nr. 1083.

1700s, probably by a wax artisan named Josef Benedikt Curiger.

Curiger was a member of a Swiss family which had a long tradition of making wax models of the body, though their wax models were originally made not for medical doctors, but as a way of praying for divine intervention. Hundreds of years ago, in some of the mountain valleys of Switzerland just as in other parts of Catholic Europe, people who were sick would buy a model of the part of the body that was diseased or injured and leave it at the altar in the local church, as a sort of offering and materialized plea for God's help. While we were down in the underground vaults looking at the wax reliefs, the archivist took me into a storage space that had stacks and stacks of boxes in it. In these boxes were the old votive offerings of body parts that had been collected from local churches. Opening one of the boxes, she showed me hundreds of wax eyes. In another box were small arms and hands, most no larger than a doll's arm. Some were made of wax, others carved out of wood or bone; some intricately painted, others just a shape that suggested what it was supposed to be. In another box there was a collection of little feet, another held fingers, and yet another, a collection of little babies. Most of these miniature figures were hundreds of years old. In those boxes were physical prayers from people who were suffering from broken bones, twisted limbs, rheumatism, unknown aches and pains, infertility, miscarriages, childhood diseases . . . people who did not have access to medical care as we know it today, and lived at a time when medicine could not solve most of their problems even if they had been able to find a doctor. Instead, they took their problems to the priest, literally. And now these problems are archived in a medical history library at the University of Zurich.

But there is something confusing about why these boxes of votives, collected from the side chapels of churches, are part of the collection of a medical history library. Or maybe not confusing but, rather, revealing. That these wax or wooden prayers for healing are stored in the same underground archive as the wax reliefs made for doctors indicates the historical (and current) traffic our bodies and diseases make between different professional and cultural domains. We can draw parallels to the prostate's appearance within anatomical knowledge, and how this coincided with a period of time when the body and its pathologies were becoming more firmly (though not exclusively, of course) the domain of medical doctors, a time when medicine was gaining ground in terms of its physical and pathological remit, and undergoing a continuous process of professionalization. This we can see when we look at how the body is represented and how it is treated, and to some extent also when we think about *who* is expected to treat disease and cure the body, where they have been taught, and what aspects of the body and the person those diseases and treatments are thought to address. I'm going to let thoughts about these aspects of medicine quietly work in the background, like a healthy, functioning prostate, as I explore prostate diagnosis and treatment practices historically and today in the next chapters.

2
What Was the Prostate?

The wax relief of the prostate in Zurich had made me wonder how medical doctors imagined and examined the prostate before the days of ultrasound, CT, and MRI scans. How did doctors discover the prostate, and how did they produce knowledge about it? Doctors have not always known what the prostate was, or even that there was an important and separate tissue with specific functions under the bladder. But by the time those wax reliefs were made, they had seen its physical contours. Yet, in the archive in Zurich, there were no boxes of little prostates collected from rural Swiss churches, even though the man who had made the wax reliefs of the prostate had probably learned his craft through carving and molding these other offerings for the lay public. At the end of the 1700s, he and artisans like him found a new market for their skills by selling reliefs in wax to medical doctors. But the prostate, as with other parts of the interior anatomy, is not as easy to see and copy as a hand or a nose meant to be left at an altar. To model it, the artisans had to employ other sources of knowledge, and often copied pictures of the human anatomy found in books at the time, in which the original pictures were drawn while watching dissections of dead bodies.[1] And in these pictures, by the 1700s, the prostate was part of the standard image of the male genital system in anatomy books. A hundred years earlier there was not even an accepted name for the prostate. And two hundred years earlier, it didn't even exist.

Well, "exist" and "exist." In some ways, this echoes the discussion of what a prostate "is." Just because the prostate did not have a name, or did not feature in standard anatomy book drawings for many centuries, that does not mean it had not caused problems. It just was not named as the source of those problems. Older men have probably always had issues with urination. There are pictures on Egyptian papyrus from the fifteenth century BCE of doctors trying to help patients urinate.[2] Hippocrates, the famous doctor from ancient Greece, wrote about urination problems.[3] Words that deal specifically with peeing like *urination*, *urine*, *urethra* and the word for the medical specialty, *urology*, all stem from the ancient Greek word to pee, *ureo*.[4] They have been used in medicine for thousands of years. But the word "prostate" has a very different history, not least because medical knowledge did not even know that men had a prostate until relatively recently. Why? Well, even though human dissections were used to learn about the body in ancient Egypt and Greece, for long periods of European history, cutting open dead human bodies to learn about anatomy was rare. At that time, much of the knowledge about the body was modeled on that produced by the Greek physician Galen in the second century. He made no mention of the prostate in his work. The prostate was not visible outside of the body, and it was not something that just happened to be exposed on a bloody battlefield or during a farming accident. No one really noticed it by chance. And, even though animal carcasses were sometimes used to extrapolate knowledge about the human body, there are significant differences between animal prostates and the human prostate.[5]

Dissection of human bodies for medical purposes started to become more widespread in European medical schools in the thirteenth and fourteenth centuries, and eventually, by the 1500s, purpose-built anatomy theaters were part of the most famous medical schools, perhaps the most well-known being the school in the Italian city of Bologna, in which dissection lectures and shows were held for both students and invited guests, sometimes set to music.[6] However, even when it did become more common to cut open dead bodies and perform public autopsies on them in the name of science, medicine, or education, it was still hard to discover the prostate. No one knew it was there, no one knew what it did, and as it was sort of the same color as the other tissue around it, most doctors, scientists, and anatomists did not see it. Leonardo da Vinci, for example, who died in 1519, missed it.[7] It was in 1536 that a physician named Niccolò Massa, working in Venice, was said to have "discovered" the prostate by writing about the existence of a gland just under the bladder. Two years later, the famous anatomist Vesalius published a sketch of this gland in the *Tabulae anatomicae sex* and later in his book *De humani corporis fabrica libri septem* (see figure 2.1).[8] This book became an early bestseller, and was a standard anatomy text, so with it, the prostate's existence was firmly established. But neither Massa nor Vesalius gave it a name; they just described or drew it. And even though it had now been "discovered,"

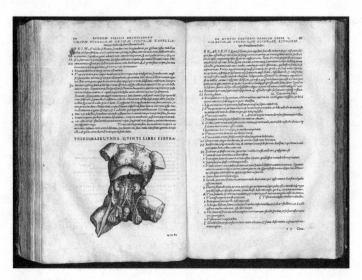

Figure 2.1

Andreas Vesalius, *De humani corporis fabrica libri septem*, 372. Published in Basel by Johannes Oporinus, 1543. From the collection of The Hagströmer Medico-Historical Library, Karolinska Institutet (KI), Stockholm, Sweden. Photo by Anna Lantz.

no one was quite sure what it did. Some people thought the gland refined the semen, others thought it made it. Some people thought it produced a fluid that moistened the urethra, still others thought it created a white fluid from the blood that would make sex more pleasurable. Its actual purpose was a mystery, though they were all close in guessing that the prostate had something to do with sex and semen.

It took more than sixty years after it was first drawn for a version of the name "prostate" to appear in European medical texts. *Prostatae* was used in print in 1600 by André du Laurens,[9] though probably other people had used this name before he wrote it down. *Prostatae* is taken from a Greek word that means roughly "the one who stands before," and probably refers to the fact that the prostate is "before" the bladder. People still were not quite sure what it did, though, and some doctors even thought it might actually be two glands, not one. This may be because the prostate has two prominent lobes or sections, but it may also be because the reproductive organs leading to it, the testicles, are paired, so it would make sense that there were two prostates, as well. Importantly, though, by the 1600s, the existence of a prostate (or two) was part of the standard core of knowledge about men's reproductive tracts; the gland had been drawn, and given a medical name: *prostatae*. By the middle of the 1700s, the word "prostate" was being used in English. And by 1800 it was generally accepted that the prostate was a single gland.[10]

Thus, by the end of the 1800s, the prostate was known to medical science, named, designated singular with discrete parts, and had a (somewhat complicated) association with sex. It was implicated in ejaculation, possibly male orgasm, and some doctors even thought that the prostate's role was to shoot sperm with such force that its impact on the cervix would cause a female orgasm.[11] The prostate was attributed an important role in reproduction, some claiming that "without it, the race would end,"[12] and, as if that wasn't enough responsibility, it was also blamed for many of men's health problems—especially those related to ageing and urination. But when it acted up, there was still a lot of uncertainty about what was actually wrong with the prostate, the causes of the problems, and how they should be fixed.[13]

Perhaps because the prostate was associated with sperm and ejaculation,[14] a common theory at the turn of the last century was that prostate problems in older men were a side effect of sowing one's wild oats in youth.[15] Sometimes doctors suspected that an older man with prostate issues had been a bit too promiscuous before settling down, or even simply masturbated too much, and these sins were now coming back to haunt him in old age.[16] Information about the patient's history of, in particular, gonorrhea, was collected when an older man presented with suspected prostate problems, and in studies that tried to find statistically relevant contributing factors to prostate diseases in larger

groups of men, gonorrhea was a very common suspect.[17] One reason for this was that, before medical
science had discovered antibiotics, a man who had con-
tracted gonorrhea in his youth would have likely had a
low-grade infection for decades by the time he reached
old age. After many, many years of untreated infection,
gonorrhea can cause scar tissue to develop inside the
urethra, scar tissue that can block the passage of urine
and produce symptoms similar to those caused by an
enlarged prostate. To doctors examining older men
with problems urinating, there sometimes seemed to
be a connection between prostate issues and gonorrhea.
It was only coincidental, but medical science did not
know that at the time (though by the beginning of the
1900s doctors were starting to debate the theory).[18] One
seemingly obvious conclusion was to say that prostate
problems might be related to sexually transmitted infections. When examining a prostate patient, therefore,
doctors also asked about the man's history of coitus
and his marital status. Medical notes about how many
patients were, for example, Catholic priests (assumed to
be celibate) and married Protestant ministers (assumed
to have been sexually active) also appear in population
studies of prostate problems at the time.[19]

By the late 1800s there were many other common
theories about what caused prostate problems. Maybe
the man had engaged in too much physical labor
involving standing. Or maybe he had spent too long at
a sedentary desk job.[20] Perhaps he had been exposed to

cold and damp. Or maybe he had done too much horse-riding. Or he had ridden in the cold and damp. . . . There were a lot of ideas about the causes of prostate problems: no one really knew for sure, and to complicate things, a large number of different names were used to describe prostate diseases. Going to the doctor for urination difficulties could get you a diagnosis of prostatitis, *prostatisme vésical*, *le prostatisme*, prostatic hypertrophy, prostatorrhoea, prostatic obstruction . . . the list continued. And, to be fair, there are still many modern terms for prostate problems. Besides the relatively common diseases like BPH and cancer, doctors can diagnose acute urinary retention (AUR); bladder outlet obstruction (BOO); or benign prostatic enlargement (BPE). Even prostatitis is still sometimes used, despite the fact that it is a very broad—and possibly often misapplied—diagnosis (see chapter 4). And I *have* heard of modern doctors who will still blame a wild youth for an older man's problems, though this is more often associated with riding motorcycles in the cold and damp than with promiscuity.

Another problem for doctors a hundred and fifty years ago was that it was really difficult to examine the prostate. This is still true, but was more so then. Think about all those pictures of the prostate in chapter 1. The technology to make those images did not exist at the end of the 1800s. Basically, doctors could ask the patient about his health, they could use their finger to try to feel the backside of the prostate through the rectum, and they could try to stick thin rods up the penis. If the patient had died, they could dissect his body. An early precursor of laparoscopy had been developed by this time: a cystoscope that was a tube with lenses which could sometimes be used to see up to the bladder, but it was a difficult and uncomfortable examination technology—especially since the instrument itself was fairly large, and there was no local anesthesia available. Many doctors (and assumedly their patients) preferred not to use it.[21] Instead, doctors would use metal sticks (sounds) to "feel" inside the urethra, which, when sharpened, could also be used to scrape away at scar tissue or other obstructions.[22] Though again, without anesthesia or antibiotics.

All this means that, at the end of the 1800s, treatments were often ineffective and sometimes downright dangerous. Nonetheless, doctors did try to find ways to help. Sometimes these treatments would involve medicines: opium, silver nitrate and belladonna suppositories, potassium iodine, potassium bromide, and ergot (a type of fungi that grows on rye).[23] Other times, they would prescribe large quantities of distilled water.[24] Many of these treatments were directed at the symptoms the man presented with, primarily urination problems, and some of the elixirs were even used to irrigate the bladder; but others, like ergot, were actually thought to shrink the prostate gland.[25] Electricity was also a trendy new technology at the time, and probes were invented which would allow doctors to give electrical shocks to the prostate by inserting one end into the rectum to direct electricity through the intestinal wall at the prostate, making a current loop with another diode placed on the testicles.[26] The goal of this treatment was also to shrink the prostate, though the inventor noted that when using the instrument, it was of vital importance to turn it off as soon as the patient started complaining of discomfort.[27]

During this time, doctors also started developing surgical methods to treat the prostate.[28] And, interestingly, there was a short time—which Björk, one of my colleagues, has studied—when castration was used to treat prostate problems. Björk's research details one brief period in the late 1800s in Northern Europe when castration was a treatment for prostate hypertrophy. While there are ontological problems with claiming that a disease we know by one name today is the same as a disease we knew by another in an earlier time period with different knowledge-making practices,[29] for ease of reference, prostate hypertrophy was a diagnosis that closely aligns with what we today call benign prostate hyperplasia, BPH. The overlap is not complete, but many of the patients' symptoms and experiences are similar. For example, men diagnosed with prostate hypertrophy tended to be older, and they presented with moderate to severe problems of urine blockage and retention. Doctors assumed that the problem was that the prostate had grown too large, or at least grown inward around the urethra, and was blocking the smooth flow of urine

out from the bladder. What caused this growth or blockage was uncertain, and thought to be possibly multifari-
ous. While today, BPH is thought to be caused by the
normal growth of the ageing prostate, in the late 1800s
there was a lot of speculation about the association with
gonorrhea scarring, mentioned above, and the clinical
observation that it seemed to blight older men who had
married a second, younger, wife and were more sexually active than was, at the time, considered fitting for a
man of their age.[30]

One way of treating prostate hypertrophy was by
poking through the tissue and creating a channel for the
urine to flow through with those sharp, metal instruments called sounds. This was often painful, and caused
additional problems. Another common treatment for
prostate hyperplasia was to use a catheter—a stick with
a hole through it, like a straw—to empty the bladder,
but catheter technology was not very highly developed,
and usually involved stiff metal tubes that made the
bladder both painful to empty and prone to infections.
That treatment was not really so different than poking
a hole through the tissue with a sharp sound. Plus, as
this was before the advent of antibiotics, urinary tract
infections, especially frequent or chronic ones triggered
by daily insertion of an inadequately cleaned catheter,
could be—and often were—life-threatening.[31] When
this was discussed in the medical literature, it would be
suggested as an option either if the patient was capable

of maintaining the necessary level of hygiene for catheterization, or if he had someone at home who could help with this, but there was a tendency to speak of the 'catheter life' as a painful, often short, and tragic way to end one's days. Some reports suggested a mortality rate as high as 8 percent within a month.[32] There were also surgical methods in use, mostly to reach and reduce the prostate tissue through the abdominal wall, but these were difficult, not necessarily successful, and also had a high mortality rate, perhaps as high as 40 percent. Against such a context, there was a real need to find an alternative treatment for prostate hypertrophy, and some doctors suggested that castration would be the best option.[33]

In the practice of removing the testicles, one can see a parallel to the way the female body was being treated by medicine at the time. Many studies have been made of the tendency to remove or otherwise treat the female sexual and reproductive organs in an attempt to cure other health problems that were plaguing the patient. Removal of the uterus and/or ovaries has been put forward as a solution to tumors and growths in the uterus, but also as a treatment for general female malaise, discontent, "hysteria," or even masturbation.[34] Björk's work on castration presents an example of medical treatment for urination problems in men consisting of removal of part of the male reproductive system, which may have been rarer. Healthy testicles were surgically removed in the hope that this would shrink the prostate.[35] She explains how, in the debates for and against the use of castration, doctors relied on an analogy between the prostate and the uterus. Because the removal of the ovaries had been an established treatment for noncancerous growths in the uterus (called uterine myoma in the literature of the time) in women, this existing treatment was an argument for castration as a cure for hypertrophy of the prostate in men. Knowledge about the female body drawn from the already established field of gynecology was thereby used as a basis to construct knowledge about the prostate. And even though the analogy between the prostate and the uterus was contested as a theory, there were nonetheless many doctors willing to test it in practice.[36]

Examples of such testing appear in the writings of British urologist Sir Henry Thompson, who claimed that both the prostate and the uterus were made up of a mass of "organic muscular fibre," and both were subjected to tumors that, in his opinion, were very similar. Thompson claimed that the uterus and the prostate could both become hypertrophied.[37] While Björk notes that the eventual rejection of castration as a cure also cast the analogy between the prostate and the uterus into question, two other colleagues I worked with, Björkman and Persson, point out that this theory was not universally discarded immediately, and that other physicians many years later could explain prostate issues as "degenerative change" similar to what one would see in an ageing uterus.[38]

Another reason why doctors were willing to try castration as a treatment at the end of the 1800s was because they had noticed that eunuchs never developed enlarged prostates, leading the medical community to suspect that there might be some connection between the testicles and prostate problems. Even though this work was being done before the establishment of our modern knowledge of hormones,[39] there was some suspicion that something was going on between the glands of the testicles and the tendency of the prostate to grow and expand pathologically.[40] Thus, theories about the curative potential of removing one or both testicles drew from existing knowledge about female bodies and on observations about bodies with prostates that had, for various reasons, been living without testicles. However, the arguments put forward for castration also relied on knowledge about nonhuman bodies, especially experimentation with castration in dogs. Dogs are one of the few animals which, when not castrated, can develop an enlarged prostate and the urination difficulties associated with it. There seemed to be evidence that castration in dogs caused the prostate to atrophy.[41] On the basis of these observations, doctors began to castrate patients in an attempt to cure prostate hypertrophy.

Perhaps not surprisingly, patient responses to the suggestion of castration were not unequivocally positive. Of course, sharp metal sticks, catheters, and the high risk of death by surgery were not attractive alternatives, nor was being unable to pee. One of my modern-day informants has told me that when he first developed an enlarged prostate and began to find himself in front of the toilet, desperate to pee and unable to get anything out, he would have gladly given up sex in exchange for a free flow of urine. Some men in the 1890s may have felt the same. But the idea of castration was met with resistance, and doctors who were trying to argue for the benefits of the procedure seemed to interpret patient protests in different ways, depending on who those patients were. Younger men who protested were considered normal. However, older men who did not want to allow themselves to be castrated were described as overly sentimental, and their protests perceived as a part of the problem.[42]

The idea that there was a connection between the *prostate* and a patient's mental and emotional health was very widespread in the nascent field of urology at the time.[43] Björkman and Persson note in their history of urology that doctors working at the beginning of the 1900s were prone to associate the prostate with both sexual (mis)behavior and mental health problems. Their material shows that the healthy prostate was understood to be "the seat of the sexual brain," at a time when doctors considered (hetero) sex within marriage to be the safest and healthiest option. Other sexual practices, like masturbation, coitus interruptus, excessive sex, and sex outside of marriage, were not only deemed morally questionable, but also associated with disease in general, and an irritated and inflamed prostate in particular.

This was explained by the theory that the prostate was being overly strained by the muscular contractions of ejaculation. However—and paradoxically—too little sex, or ungratified sexual desire, were also suspected of causing an inflamed prostate. . . . One could not win, unless one was having a respectable amount of (hetero) sex within marriage.[44]

At the same time, there was a theory that the enlarged prostate itself could lead to increased sexual desire, and that it was often the *cause* of older men suffering from "amorous senility," i.e., courting women much younger than themselves. The debate about whether the diseased prostate was the cause or the effect of inappropriate sexual behavior may seem entertaining today, but if we read it through the lens of history, we can see that these descriptions of the healthy prostate were actually descriptions of the physicians' own ideas about "respectable" sexual behavior for men of their age, class, and social position.[45]

Björkman and Persson's work demonstrates that the prostate's health and sexual behavior was thought to both impact and reflect on a man's *mental* health in European and North American medical literature at the turn of the last century, and be used as a diagnosis when a "man had overstepped the bounds of healthy, normal and moral sexuality. As a result, [the man] became vulnerable, weak, impotent, irrational and even insane."[46] Doctors thought that the inflamed prostate could call forth hypochondria, neurasthenia, hallucinations, and suicidal tendencies, and be a cause of memory loss, lack of concentration, lowered intellectual capacities, and insomnia. It was not clear how this was happening, though different theories existed, including that there might be some sort of "internal secretion" from the prostate that exerted "a direct influence on the psychic state of the brain."[47] But, as with the discussion of sexuality, Björkman and Persson point out that these diagnoses were simultaneously descriptions of a normative masculinity.[48] They associated disease in men with characteristics typically assigned to the era's understanding of femininity, like weakness, vulnerability, irrationality, and insanity.[49] The weak and diseased prostate was associated with a weak and diseased masculinity.

Because of these associations, a man at the turn of the last century who could not urinate had multiple reasons to be concerned about his prostate. His need to urinate, of course, was pressing first and foremost. But he also needed to be concerned about his relationship to social norms of sexuality and masculinity. Likewise, the medical doctor he consulted was interested in the discussions of treatment options, and survival rates, but also curious about causes and, if following the advice of medical literature for the period, would have been encouraged to search for those causes in things like the man's marital status, sexual practices, and professional occupation.

The patients and their doctors were not the only social actors interested in the ageing prostate. Wider society was also concerned with the health of (some) older men,[50] and knowledge about the prostate, its problems, treatments, and side effects, and how these related to other aspects of life, became a point of discussion outside the clinic, as well. Examples of these connections can be found in the speculation about the types of men and types of jobs associated with prostate problems that featured in medical literature from the time.[51] And even once the direct connection between sexual mores, masculinity, and prostate health tapered off as the twentieth century progressed, certain actors in society continued to have an interest in the prostate for reasons other than purely urological concerns. For example, while I was going through the material from the Semmelweis archive, seated in their wood-paneled reading room in Budapest, I came across a text from 1936 in which a then renowned urologist addressed the medical directors of the American Association of Life Insurance providers, speaking about new surgical procedures that could both lower the number of patients who died from surgery and also provide surgical relief to men before their prostate problems became so advanced that they were forced to stop working.[52] His lecture spoke volumes about the commercial interests that wanted to maintain a healthy, male, working population as long as possible, interests which then translated into reasons to care about the development of prostate problems and surgical procedures to cure them. And, of course, since the prostate was a source of potential disease and death, its rates of pathology and the age men usually incurred such problems was of interest to life insurers, in particular,[53] who are naturally interested in the health and mortality rate of those who buy their policies. In the context of a lecture for the life insurers, the prostate became a scientific object of concern beyond the medical clinic: of interest to external actors, including the directors of companies who wanted to ensure (and insure) their healthy, male workforce.

An Evolving Prostate

Castration, at least the surgical version, was eventually abandoned as a treatment for prostate hypertrophy. Social and medical reasons were intertwined in its eventual disappearance. Patient resistance was certainly one contributing factor, but so too was the fact that few patients showed long-term improvement after castration.[54] And, importantly, technological innovation also changed the treatment options available; catheter technology improved, especially when better hygiene methods were developed, reducing infection and death rates. And new surgical procedures had better survival rates—sometimes even better success rates.[55] Then there was the problem that mental distress was specifically associated with the removal of one or both testicles, as doctors began to report that some male patients developed psychological problems after castration.[56] This was slightly unexpected, because it meant that, in the late 1800s, removal of the ovaries was being used as a treatment *for* psychological problems in women, but removal of the testicles was thought to *cause* them in men, disrupting the contemporary parallel theorization between the treatment of male and female reproductive organs.[57]

Today, rather than *physically* castrating patients, hormonal methods have been developed to treat specific prostate problems: a development which can trace its inspiration to the experiments with castration at the turn of the last century.[58] In the 1930s and 1940s, doctors began to use testosterone and estrogen in different combinations to treat "prostatism," as it was then being called, and by the 1970s and 1980s, medical science had moved to trials of anti-androgens and progestins. Some of these treatments actually alleviated patient symptoms, especially problems with urine flow, even though many of them had severe side effects like vertigo, shivering, tiredness, loss of libido, and impotence.[59] They were not considered completely successful. They did, however, set the stage for some of the medicines used to treat the prostate today. For example, one of the current treatments for prostate cancer involves hormone therapy, and some of the modern medicines for benign prostate hyperplasia manipulate levels of certain testosterone metabolites (like 5-alpha-dihydrotestosterone).

But what does this tell us about the prostate, as the question is framed both in chapter 1 and here? What "was" the prostate, and what "is" the prostate? These questions are intimately connected to how we know it and what we associate it with. How are our medical and social imaginaries[60] entangled? And how does this entanglement impact on anatomical, diagnostic, and treatment options? For example, at the turn of the last century the prostate was associated with sexuality and mental health even if it was unclear how, specifically, those associations worked. Was an enlarged and diseased prostate the cause of sexual excess, or was sexual excess the cause of disease in the prostate? Was a diseased prostate the cause of nervousness and insanity, or were mental excesses from office work or stress triggers for prostate disease? It wasn't clear. But despite this uncertainty, the association between them was so strong in the medical discourse that the prostate could be used to speak about values and norms as well as about health and disease. In this sense, the prostate and its health became a stand-in for conversations about socially appropriate sexuality, health, masculinity, and vigor. Aspects of a man's identity could be used to discuss and diagnose his prostate, but so could his prostate be used to diagnose his identity.

In the historical examples in this chapter, the prostate appears with different cultural contours depending on what it is associated with and how it is imagined to function. At various times it has been: a gland that was possibly impacted by the shift to sedentary office work that many men experienced in urban areas during the late 1800s;[61] a gland that could become 'bothered' by the weather, especially the cold and the damp;[62] a gland that was blamed for tormenting and torturing men with pain, urination troubles, infection, and often death, either directly or through the side effects of treatment. It was also a part of the ejaculatory system, becoming a gland that produced the male orgasm[63] and maybe even enabled female orgasm,[64] and thus fertilization (at a time when some thought female orgasm was necessary for conception);[65] a gland that influenced how sexually active older men were, prompting them to chase younger women in inappropriate ways;[66] a gland that became diseased because of this sort of "inappropriate" behavior, thus becoming something within the body that was enlarged and diseased as a result of particular behaviors.[67] And given that there was uncertainty about the relationship between prostate problems and gonorrhea, the prostate was also, discursively, a location of sexually transmitted infection and the moral insinuations associated with it at the end of the 1800s.[68] These, together with theories about how the prostate and the uterus were homologous, led to castration being a possible solution to its problems, reflecting how social and cultural elements that are part of various definitions of our body's anatomy can have very important implications for how we and the medical community imagine potential treatments.

This is not the same as saying that our cultural imaginary is what makes the prostate. For example, by saying the prostate was not present in Europe before the 1500s, I am not suggesting that the tissue did not exist, or that it did not cause problems as it became diseased or enlarged. Again, urination problems in older men have always existed. But until the prostate became an object of knowledge and was named, it was not possible to associate these problems to the gland. The same goes for that association with "inappropriate sexual behavior" in the older male made at the end of the 1800s. That we no longer associate such behavior with the enlarged prostate, but did only 150 years ago, shows how useful it can be to study these various definitions of what the prostate "is" if we want to understand cultural contexts and values, and possibly to see remnants of them in our understanding of the prostate today. We can use these definitions of the prostate and its diseases to refract[69] and make visible cultural norms, and help us to understand what values and expectations we placed on bodies with prostates in the past. And still place on them today. In these ways, the prostate "is" slightly different things, and does different things, throughout history. Even if there is an underlying illness and problem with urination that may be similar for those experiencing symptoms across time and in different cultural contexts, explanations can vary, and those different explanations can, together with technological and medical knowledge, influence what sort of treatment options are imaginable.[70]

The "is" of the prostate, today and in the past, also reveals a flickering element of absence/presence. Remember the film I mentioned at the beginning of chapter 1, made as a response to the absence of knowledge about the prostate in younger men even as its presence as an imaginary harbinger of cancer and death was ever-present. That film addressed the question of what the prostate "is" by making it present in a couple of very specific ways. We used illustrations to make it visible on the screen. We simply drew it, but there are many different visualization technologies available to produce images of the prostate today, the choice of which contributes to how the prostate "looks" to the viewer, but also indicates which care trajectory the patient is in, and produces images that are useful in different ways to those different trajectories. In the film, we used the drawings and narrative to position the prostate in the viewer's body and relate it to other parts of the male reproductive system, which gave it a presence in the viewer's physical anatomy but also a presence in the process of ejaculation, anchoring it as an important and healthy part of an activity their body was already engaged in, and creating a healthy presence for it rather than just the impending doom of prostate cancer. But then, at the end of the film, the narrator tells the viewer that most of the time the prostate just sits quietly in the body, doing what it is supposed to do and not making itself known; this lets the prostate as a medical object and a figure of thought slink back into absence, or into the phenomenological silence[71] that the healthy body is thought to have.

This, however, is a book about the prostate, and much of its "presence" is associated with disease. Thus, the following chapters are going to trace how it is present within the contours of disease today; how the "is" of the modern prostate is useful for understanding and refracting the norms and values applied to bodies with prostates now, just as they were in the past. Until, of course, the final chapter, in which the prostate is both absent, physically, after surgical removal and present, culturally, in the effects its absence has on the body, and the psychological and social implications that absence has for the men who are living without it. After removal, the prostate sometimes becomes more present than ever before . . . but more on that later. In the next few chapters, I will look at modern medical practices for diagnosing the prostate and determining what it "is": how the prostate as a medical object has become an explanatory factor in many different medical discourses today.

3
Contours of the Prostate Today

Conjure up the image of a group of older men riding racing bikes through the American Southwest. Cut to a scene of them resting at the rim of the Grand Canyon, drinking refreshingly from large water bottles. Cut to another scene of those same men kayaking on a wild river . . . and then to another of them enjoying drinks at an outdoor café . . . and then sleeping, undisturbed, through the night.[1]

Or, more depressingly, imagine a man being constantly bothered by a nagging need to go pee while playing golf. Then, cut to him, sitting totally boxed in, stuck in a nightmare traffic jam . . . having to go pee. And then, waking up in the middle of the night . . . to go pee.[2]

These are some examples of pharmaceutical advertising imagery used to promote medicines that can treat prostate problems, images that show men (often white, often middle- class,[3] often older, but usually very active) doing things that one would not want to interrupt with frequent trips to the bathroom, like outdoor sports, driving, or chess.[4]

Older men with urination problems are sometimes (often?) diagnosed as having an enlarged prostate, also known as lower urinary tract symptoms secondary to benign prostate hyperplasia (LUTS/BPH). The symptoms that produced the prostatic hypertrophy in the 1800s would, today, probably indicate LUTS/BPH. This chapter examines diagnostic tests recommended in the clinical guidelines for LUTS/BPH,[5] looking at each sort of examination in the order they are suggested to see how the body, and especially the prostate, becomes an object and cause of the disease. I suggest[6] that, by thinking about something (a prostate, BPH, blocked urine, for example), we make invisible the social and technological contingencies that produce that thing in very specific ways. And, just as in the historical material discussed above, the scientific and the social become blurred, but the diagnostic practices hide that blurring.

But first, some background: LUTS/BPH is a disease of the enlarged prostate. For some men, the prostate starts to enlarge at around fifty years of age; for others, not until they are seventy, or older. It is a normal development, but this normal growth can cause problems with urination because, when the prostate gets larger, it may also start to block the urethra. By the age of seventy, 75 percent of men will have BPH symptoms, i.e., problems urinating.[7] It is when the prostate begins to block the flow of urine through the urethra that the enlargement of the prostate becomes a problem, which means the prostate's normal resumption of growth becomes pathological.[8] Today, this problem is often treated with pharmaceuticals, including hormone-regulating compounds, but other methods are also used to reduce or destroy the regrowth zones of the prostate in hope of releasing pressure on the urethra and facilitating urination; these include microwave treatments and electrical heating, and a fairly common method called transurethral resection of the prostate (TURP), where a doctor uses a tool inserted through the urethra to cut out prostate tissue from the inside.[9] But before any of this can be done, the man experiencing urination problems must be diagnosed.

It is that diagnostic practice I am looking at here. At the same time, I will continue to unpack what the prostate "is" by looking how we gain knowledge about it today. Given that the prostate primarily appears when it is the source of trouble—when it is interrupting long bike rides, kayaking trips, fly-fishing, and chess games— this question becomes: What is done to diagnose a diseased, troublesome prostate? Diagnosis of prostate problems involves complex practices that produce specific outcomes. Some of these practices are related to how we are in the world and with other people; they are social. By making those social practices invisible through testing and diagnostic tools, they are bracketed.[10] To open that up,[11] as in the historical chapter, I will also be pointing out where and how social expectations and norms appear and shape the medical practices of understanding the diseased prostate.

LUTS/BPH: When the Prostate Grows and Blocks Urination

LUTS/BPH is one of the most common diseases of the ageing prostate, along with cancer. In this diagnosis, urination problems become prostate problems as they are described, measured, and understood by the doctor, and assigned to a disease category called LUTS, Lower Urinary Tract Symptoms. These symptoms are generally associated with men over fifty,[12] even though recent guidelines from the American Urology Association (AUA) include men as young as forty-five,[13] and older women also can present with lower urinary tract symptoms. In fact, one study has suggested that older women have lower urinary tract symptoms more frequently than men.[14] However, in the discussion of LUTS/BPH, lower urinary tract symptoms are ascribed to men over fifty, and most often to men significantly older.

In the diagnosis of LUTS/BPH, a distinction is made between *bothersome* lower urinary tract symptoms and *non-bothersome* lower urinary tract symptoms. Just because a patient seeks help from his doctor for urinary tract symptoms does not necessarily mean that he is suffering from *bothersome* lower urinary tract symptoms: that is, defined as bothersome enough to warrant treatment, not just bothersome enough to prompt a visit to a doctor. The literature suggests that—particularly now, with the increasing awareness of prostate cancer and its screening methods—more men are likely to seek medical attention for changes in urinary patterns or other, diffuse, lower urinary tract symptoms, but that in some of these cases the best course of action is to test for cancer, reassure the patient that they are cancer-free, talk about changes to the urinary tract associated with ageing, and then suggest lifestyle changes (reduced consumption of liquids in the evening, for example), rather than initiating medical intervention.[15] But how does one know when bothersome is bothersome enough to do something more? Officially, determining the level of bother is done by an evaluation of the patient's medical history (questions about the nature and duration of the lower urinary tract symptoms); their sexual function; their general health (both as a contributing factor for lower urinary tract symptoms and as a determining factor for potential invasive procedures); a review of the patient's current medications (some of which can contribute to urinary disturbances); prior surgical procedures that could affect urination; and weight, physical exercise, diet, etc.[16] Together, these give a picture of the man's overall state of health and the state of his urinary tract.

How Bothersome Is It?

But, still, how does one know when this bother is just too bothersome? The best way is probably to ask—and a series of questions (the Symptoms Score Index) has been used, and improved upon over several decades; these

questions produce a symptom score reflecting voiding and storage, and ascertain specifically how bothersome the symptoms are, and how much they affect the
patient's quality of life. These scores, combined with
the physical examination, a frequency volume chart,
and a peak flow rate recording, among other things, all
say something about specific urination practices. And
together they produce the diseased prostate as a knowledge object.[17]

The Symptoms Score Index is a standard set of questions used in both North America and around the world.
The first standardized questionnaire for lower urinary
tract symptoms was published in 1976.[18] Since then the
questions have been fine-tuned and developed further
and, above all, a question about how bothersome the
symptoms are and how they affect the man's quality of
life has been added and validated. The questions in this
survey ask about how frequently the patient has been
able to empty their bladder completely, how often they
need to urinate, if they have to stop and restart during
urination, if they are able to postpone urination when
necessary, if they need to strain to initiate it, and how
often they need to get up to go to the bathroom during the night. The questionnaire also includes a subjective question about how the patient would perceive
their current urination problems, should these continue
indefinitely. The individual scores for each of these
questions are then added up, and the patient's experience of bother is assigned a number.[19]

During the 1990s, studies were done to see how the symptom scores generated by the questionnaire correlated to the "bothersome" question. Men in many different countries were asked, and their responses were compared.[20] There were not always direct geographical correlations (one study found that men in Scotland reported fewer symptoms, but just as much bother, as men in Minnesota,[21] for example) but the bothersome level and symptom severity did seem to generally align,[22] and could therefore be added to the diagnostic toolbox. It became apparent that different sorts of symptoms produced different levels of bother (voiding problems generally seemed to be less bothersome than storage problems, except that men ranked the posturination dribble the single most bothersome symptom).[23] It also became clear that the initial experience of bother at the time of the first visit could determine future care trajectories, and that bothersome levels generally decreased after surgery or other treatments,[24] so this questionnaire was also used as a way of determining the success of treatment. Studies have returned to these questions, reevaluating and revalidating them on a regular basis to confirm their continued reliability, and the survey[25] is still a basic starting point in the diagnostic procedure for LUTS/BPH.[26]

A Swedish scientific literature review of BPH[27] mentions that the numerical scale assigned to the symptoms and bothersome questions gives little or no diagnostic information except that the patient has a disease of the lower urinary tract. This report went so far as to suggest that "it is important to keep in mind that high symptom points are not the same as a large degree of bother, as not all symptoms are equally bothersome."[28] This is an interesting point, because, as a Swedish urologist I interviewed said, "That questionnaire is designed to give a high score." However, even though there are sometimes questions about the usefulness of this survey and its relevance outside of the North American context, the questionnaire is widely used, has been translated into many languages, and carries with it the authority of endorsements by professional organizations like the American Urological Association, the European Association of Urology, and the World Health Organization.

The questions enroll the patient and his experiences as a source of knowledge, as he is expected to answer them himself, rather than having a medical professional do this for him. The doctor is supposed simply to take his answers and translate them into a numerical value for his lower urinary tract symptoms. The point of a validated survey which translates answers into numbers—into objective, quantified knowledge, inscribed and transferable[29]—is to remove the doctor's subjective influence from the phenomenon of understanding the lower urinary tract symptoms. But it does not remove the doctor entirely. The doctor is still there as the initiator of the survey, the recipient of the answers, and the representative of medical expertise which justifies the use of the questionnaire. The survey questions also grant legitimacy to the urology experts and organizations, and their ownership of the lower urinary tract symptoms as a urology problem, by using their approved questionnaire. The man's bothersome urination becomes a urology concern and not a diet, drinking, cardiovascular, or ageing concern (which some studies suggest it might be).[30] The questionnaire and the very name, lower urinary tract symptoms, categorize a collection of problems into one term, collapsing a heterogeneous assembly of symptoms into a single, bounded category. This process was initially necessary for the construction of the questionnaire (deciding which symptoms would be asked about, like frequency of and difficulties with urination, while eliminating others, like dribbling and leaking), and those decisions are reenacted each time the survey is used.

This is the first place where the social appears and then disappears (is bracketed) in the diagnosis of an enlarged prostate. The practices of urination that are asked about in the questionnaire are produced in a social context, a social context that is then bracketed by the numbers used to describe it. Patient experiences and social expectations are embedded into each question. For example, the first question asks about how often the patient has the sensation of not emptying his bladder entirely, which assumes that the patient knows what this sensation feels like and can differentiate it from having a completely empty bladder. Question number two assumes that urinating more frequently than once every two hours is not normal, which also carries with it the assumption that normal, daytime urination occurs less frequently than every two hours and, in questions three and four, that normal, healthy urination involves being able to start, stop, and postpone urination easily rather than running to the bathroom or standing at the urinal, straining to initiate flow. Likewise, as in question seven, there is an assumed normality about the number of times a person should have to wake up to go to the bathroom in the middle of the night.

It may seem uncontroversial to make these assumptions about urinary practices, and many (most?) people do or would want to be able to share them, myself included. But my point is that there are presumptions about normality behind them, which is always a clue that social practices and structures are also involved. For example, defining normal frequency as less than once every two hours is, in the medical literature, sometimes associated with difficulties for the man to participate in social activities like movies and concerts. However, these events are also organized around collective understandings of "normal" attention spans and "normal" urination practices, normal behaviors that are not universal. Small children do not practice them, pregnant women do not have them, and, the survey would imply, older men might not, either. But the physical world, with limited public toilet facilities, underwear instead of absorbent pads or catheters, two-hour movies, evenings at the theater with one intermission and limited toilet facilities, and infamous 18-hole golf courses, is built for people with "normal" but perhaps not statistically average, and certainly not universal, urination practices. That is the "normal" reflected in the assumptions behind some of these questions.[31]

The particular cultural assumptions behind the concept of normal urination in relation to an enlarged prostate can be seen most clearly in the articles about the often-cited Olmsted County Study initiated in the late 1980s: a large-scale research project that tried to determine the rate of LUTS/BPH in a "normal" population by surveying men in Olmsted County, Minnesota, USA. This survey is frequently referred to in literature[32] about LUTS/BPH because it is thought to give some sort of baseline idea of how many men can be expected to develop enlarged prostates, and at what age. The survey was based on questions about behavior; these questions assumed that certain behaviors would be normal for the men being questioned, and would indicate if their urination was so abnormal that it forced them to change their behavior or impacted on their daily activities, psychological health, or sexual activities. It was a population-based study, which means that many men were surveyed over a longer period of time; it was also used as one of the data baselines to rank the degree of bother men experienced from their urinary changes for a series of activities the researchers thought were standard, everyday activities for the men in Olmsted, Minnesota, thirty years ago. These included drinking fluids before travel, drinking fluids before going to bed, driving for two hours without stopping, getting enough sleep at night, going to places that might not have a toilet, playing sports outdoors, and going to movies, shows, church, etc.[33]

I am not disagreeing with the assertion that these activities could be considered normal for men in Olmsted County in the late 1980s. But by turning them into standard knowledge about LUTS/BPH, those assumptions about what is normal social behavior associated with urination are being bracketed. Then, as bracketed assumptions, they are also found in the way the questions are worded in current versions of the questionnaire, and made more invisible as answers are quantified and turned into a numerical score. That numerical score is important both for determining what sorts of management techniques will be appropriate for the patient and for deciding if treatments are working or not. But it is the *score* that is used, a score—a number denoting diagnosis—that brackets off much more than practices of administrating a symptoms questionnaire; it is a score which makes invisible the assumptions about normal urination practices and the social contexts of which they are a part. As it becomes a frequently cited study and a basis for eventual diagnostic routines in countries around the world, the normal of Olmsted, Minnesota becomes translated into the normal for many other populations.[34]

Isolating the Problem, Producing a Prostate

Once the patient has been determined to have bothersome LUTS/BPH, he enters into a further series of diagnostic tests. Aside from the infamous (often dreaded, frequently joked about) digital rectal examination, which will be discussed below, there is also a separate, more general physical examination which doctors are encouraged to conduct on patients presenting for lower urinary tract symptoms: the patient is asked about his medical history, then the doctor examines the bladder, perineum, and lower limbs. The doctor is supposed to assess the suprapubic area for bladder distension, see and feel the perineum for motor and sensory function, and check the functions of the lower limbs,[35] all with the goal of eliminating the possibility of these problems on the path to finding the issue with the prostate.

When the doctor is done examining the position of the bladder, the perineum, and the lower limbs, declaring them healthy, these anatomical organs are no longer under suspicion. The purpose of this examination is to rule out bladder, muscular, or neurological causes of lower urinary tract symptoms. Because of this, there is one other organ that is absent, yet present, in the physical examination: the prostate. Even though the prostate is not an anatomical part being seen or felt in this first, physical, examination, its presence within the unspoken discourse of LUTS/BPH as a potential, possibly even likely, candidate for the cause of the problem means that it directs the examination's attempts to rule out other urinary tract issues. It is not felt, physically, but it influences the trajectory of further examinations. Provided that the examination determines that these parts of the body are "healthy," these anatomical parts are then discarded from the scenario—they are normal, unmarked, uninteresting. The suspicions about the prostate remain, and further examinations of the lower urinary tract symptoms are initiated.

Frequency Volume Chart: When You Gotta Go . . .

At this point, patients are often given the frequency volume chart, where they are asked to keep a diary with time of urination and volume voided, often for at least one forty-eight-hour period. This chart is supposed to be particularly useful for measuring nocturia (frequent urination during the night), but it can be used in other ways, too, not least because it gives an indication of how much liquid is being expelled, and thereby also how much liquid is being consumed. According to AUA guidelines, excessive fluid intake is "common in the ageing male,"[36] and if this is the source of the LUTS problem, then reducing liquid consumption (particularly alcohol, especially in the evening) can be a solution. Perhaps even more so than with the formulation of the questions for the symptom survey, ideas about the normality of the frequency and volume of urination (and about liquid intake and alcohol consumption) are bracketed by this chart. What is considered normal intake is spoken about as normal output—urination, both during the day and during the night.

Assumptions about normal urination also appear in the built environment that the men's bodies are moving around in, especially public toilet infrastructures which are not organized around frequent toilet visits (i.e., on airline flights or train trips, at movies, concerts, and sports events). In some cases, the gradually increasing dissonance between a man's changing urination patterns and the previously unnoticed, unmarked public toilet infrastructure may be what triggered him to seek medical help in the first place. The decision to see the doctor may have been precipitated by clashes between his changing bodily needs and the systems and expectations for which public urination facilities were designed, as well as raised eyebrows in the face of frequent urination. Such changes in his body may also be exaggerated by external factors, like oversized drinks, complaining partners whose sleep is disturbed, long bus rides, and outdoor activities far from lavatories. All of these elements, visible and invisible, are bracketed by the frequency volume chart and its quantification of the patient's urination.

The numbers produced by the frequency volume chart describe and inscribe[37] how often and how much a man urinates. They quantify it, giving a number that is transportable from a general practitioner's office to a urology clinic, and comparable over time or to other men. But they are numbers that describe an action. How much liquid is the man passing? How often is he urinating? The frequency volume chart says something about practice. Yet, within the framework of diagnostic guidelines for LUTS/BPH, the numbers work together to say with one voice—or, rather, a set of numbers— something about the man's lower urinary tract symptoms, and eventually his prostate.

Flow Rate Recording: No Longer Writing One's Name in the Snow

Another diagnostic tool that potential LUTS/BPH patients may encounter are technologies for measuring the rate of urine flow during actual urination. There are many different varieties of flow rate machines that divide volume by time (milliliters/second), and the measurement can even be done (or at least estimated) by simply clocking the urination and then dividing the time by the volume (seconds/deciliters), although this latter method does not say anything about changes in flow rate during the course of urination. Many of the more advanced machines will produce graphs or charts of the flow rate which show peaks and dips, and a final number that is thought to indicate the probability of whether or not the patient is urodynamically obstructed.[38] The flow rate test and its machine together produce another number that is translatable and transportable outside of the clinic and through time. In fact, this number, called the Qmax or the peak urination flow, is one of the most commonly discussed results of the test, and, like many of the other diagnostic technologies, it is used both during the diagnosis process and as a measurement of treatment success (figure 3.1).

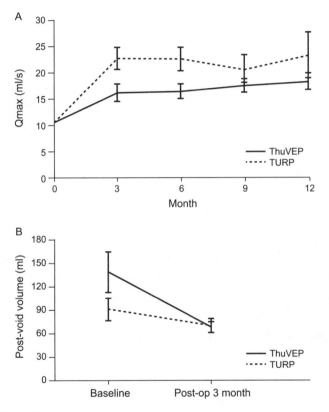

Figure 3.1
Ching-Hsin Chang, Tzu-Ping Lin, and Yen-Hwa Chang, "Vapoenucleation of the Prostate Using a High-Power Thulium Laser: A One-Year Follow-Up Study," figure 3, *BMC Urology* 15 (2015): 40. Creative Commons Attribution 4.0 International license.

However, the flow rate test is not able to diagnose an enlarged prostate or its potential shrinkage unequivocally on its own. For example, a low Qmax, meaning that the man urinates slowly, can indicate a problem, but does not determine if that problem is caused by an obstruction in the urethra (perhaps from the prostate) or a decreased detrusor contractibility (the muscle that empties the bladder).[39] Additionally, there is a significant amount of "intra-individual variability," meaning that the same man can urinate at different rates at different times of the day, and since the rate of flow is volume-dependent, the AUA suggests that at least two flow rates for a urination with a volume more than 150 milliliters should be obtained during diagnosis.[40]

The medical term "intra-individual variability" is used here to define variations in flow rate for a man at a certain period in time—maybe his stream is stronger in the morning, or perhaps after several large glasses of water. But flow rate does actually vary, normally, with age, as well. For those of us in northern climates, it may come as no surprise that it is easier for a young man to write his name in the snow than for an older man. That seems to be part of our cultural imaginary. One of the urologists I spoke with here in Sweden said that a large part of his consultation dialogues aimed to get men to understand that they were not going to be urinating with the same strength at seventy as they did at seventeen. Intra-individual variability can have different timescales.

But,[41] if a man merely complained that his stream was not as strong as it used to be, this complaint could warrant concern but would not generate a Qmax number interpreted as a pathological flow rate. Without the machine and the Qmax number, the flow rate would still be embedded in the man's descriptions of urination problems. However, by turning the flow into a flow rate recording and the production of a Qmax number, a numerical value is produced that can be used to say something about the possibility of obstruction or muscular problems, and a treatment's potential success or failure. Here, too, potential treatment practices are discursively present, albeit silently in the background, which strengthens the potential relationship between a Qmax number and the diagnostic practices for enlarged prostates. And it transfers the source of knowledge about a flow from the man who is urinating to the technology producing a statement about it.

Additionally, this Qmax number, like the scores from the questionnaire and the frequency volume chart, indicates something about the urination—the highest speed of the urine flow, how fast the man is expelling it. But in the use of the Qmax as an indicator of obstruction, something else happens. The number is asked to say something about the physical anatomy, again turning a description of a practice into an indicator of a pathologized anatomy, and into speculation about obstructions of the urethra.

Digital Rectal Examination: That Gloved Finger

I have a relative who was diagnosed with a bothersome, enlarged prostate many years ago and, for various reasons, chose to have his prostate reduced surgically through the urethra rather than treated with medications. He is quite satisfied with the results of the procedure, but every year he goes back to his urologist for a checkup. I was talking about this with him and he said that during his most recent checkup, which included a digital rectal examination (when the doctor inserts a finger into the rectum to feel the prostate's size and texture), his doctor had inserted two fingers instead of one.

"Afterwards, I asked him why he had used two fingers, since he normally doesn't," my relative told me. "And you know what he said?"

"No," I answered, falling blindly for the bait.

"Because he wanted a second opinion!" He burst into laughter. I laughed along politely, but my mind started swirling with thoughts about the prostate, and what methods and techniques are used to create knowledge about it.

All of the examinations I have detailed so far have measured urination. But my relative's joke was about an examination that actually feels the prostate. It is this examination in the diagnostic process which finally "knows" the prostate. (As if "knows" was any simpler to use than "is.") The prostate becomes the object of knowledge in a palatable way that is stationary or stable;

it is a thing, rather than an action. The rectal examination is feeling an entity, not measuring a process like urination, or a collection of experiences, like the symptom scales.

Besides checking for the size of the prostate, the rectal examination also notes the tone of the sphincter, but primarily, when a doctor is presented with a suspected LUTS/BPH patient, the rectal examination is used to determine the size, consistency, shape, and presence or absence of nodules suggesting cancer.[42] Before the PSA test was well-established as an indicator of prostate cancer (I will discuss this below), the digital rectal examination was the primary method of finding prostate cancer, and it is still useful for discovering tumors that are large enough to be palpable. The rectal examination lets the doctor feel if the prostate is abnormally shaped or bumpy, indicating possible cancerous growth,[43] and it is used by both general practitioners and urologists.[44] Not all general practitioners in Sweden have access to a transrectal ultrasound machine, so here most men are first given a manual rectal examination at their regular health clinic before being referred to a urologist and examined again, both manually and by ultrasound.[45]

During the rectal examination, the doctor's fingers rely on sensory medical knowledge about what a prostate should feel like, gleaned from previous examinations they have done, discussions with teachers and experts, medical literature, simulator training, and anatomical models. This medical knowledge gives legitimacy to rectal examination practice, but there are aspects of the prostate knowledge that are slightly unstable; for example, its size is both established *and* called into question. As the American Urology Association states, "The [rectal examination] estimation of prostate volume has been shown to be inaccurate when compared to transrectal ultrasound. The volumes of small prostates tend to be overestimated and those of large glands tend to be underestimated."[46] It is not easy to gauge the size of the prostate with one's fingers, but this is the first way it is "measured."

Results of the rectal examination bracket concerns about cancer and the notion about a normal "feel" of the prostate. The rectal examination also brackets the understandings of a man and his experiences of this examination. It is a quick one, often over in less than a minute, but many men dread and avoid it, possibly because of cultural associations of anal penetration with homosexuality.[47] It can also, on occasion, hurt. Many men find it unpleasant.

One of my colleagues, a medical anthropologist, has studied the way intimate examinations are taught to medical students in Sweden.[48] While her focus has been on gynecological examinations,[49] in the context of our research project Gleisner observed how the rectal examination was taught to medical students, and compared this with how the bimanual pelvic examination (an equally invasive and potentially uncomfortable gynecological practice) was taught.[50] The differences were striking. While the gynecological examination was embedded in lectures and course literature about care for the patient's discretion, respect for and wonder at their reproductive anatomy, and concern over any potential emotional history of abuse or fear the patient might be carrying with them into this intimate and invasive examination, the prostate examination was taught and conducted as a straightforward, disease-focused process which the patient (and, to a large extent, the medical student) was expected to perform in a perfunctory way, with little regard for how patient or doctor was experiencing the examination and even less respect for, or wonder and amazement at, the anatomy and what it can do.[51] And in fact, just writing that sentence sounds odd—wonder and amazement at the prostate and the anal canal are hardly what one expects to find in general, but specifically not in a medical examination. Nor does one think of patients undergoing digital rectal examination as a group that would demand gentle, more respectful care. This group, often consisting of older men, are generally perceived as the standard, normal, patients for whom medical care is designed. We don't imagine them to be a group prone to have experienced abuse or traumatic events in the past which could impact on their patient experiences in the present. We imagine urology patients and gynecology patients very differently, and those imaginaries contribute to the types of care practices patients encounter in the clinic: care practices which bracket our presumptions about what a male patient is and what that masculinity needs, wants, or can put up with. And patients pick up on this. The encounter with the urologist is often treated as "men's business" and very matter-of-fact,[52] without the doctor thinking about how the patient might be feeling, and without the patient expressing those feelings to the doctor.

Our imaginaries may not be serving us well, though. When I was talking with an American urologist about how he learned his rectal examination techniques in medical school, he said that he *had* actually been able to practice on a volunteer patient during the course, but that it had been a straightforward exercise. He had put his finger up the rectum and felt around until the volunteer confirmed that he had felt the prostate, then he had pulled out his finger, and was done. It wasn't until much later, after years of examining patients, that he had gradually changed his examination techniques and demeanor, taking time to first listen to and engage with the barrage of jokes he had heard a hundred times before ("Are you going to take me out to dinner afterwards, Doc?"), then encouraging the patient to relax, finding ways to reduce the tension in the room and respect the vulnerability the patient might be feeling. These shifts in practice made the examination easier, and probably better.

The jokes this urologist hears from his patients, the one my relative told me about his examination, and the prevalence of the rectal examination as a staple of

Hollywood comedies and stand-up routines about getting older, can all be read to indicate the physical, but also the social, discomfort associated with the rectal examination. If we understand humor as a well-known coping mechanism, obviously the rectal examination is having an impact on patients, and looms large as an unwelcome part of men's healthcare—for young and old alike. The jokes may be a way of making light of a situation many patients find unpleasant and scary, in contexts where humor is exposing a tension that medical care practices could address. One could envision a urological care environment that doesn't expect stoic masculinity but allows for patient vulnerability—and a medical education that produces doctors comfortable with dealing with that vulnerability from the get-go.

PSA (Prostate-Specific Antigen) Levels and Size

Another—and, according to some guidelines, perhaps the most accurate—way of measuring the size of the prostate, though without touching, feeling, or seeing it, is the prostate-specific antigen (PSA) test.[53] The PSA test changes in relation to when it is used and what it is used for. This test is often, and somewhat controversially, used for testing and screening for prostate cancer (see chapter 5).[54] It is also used after prostate cancer treatments to test if the cancer has come back. In that context, it produces fear but also promises relief (engaging the desire to be declared cancer-free), and therewith the hope for normality. The PSA test can indicate disease, and it can hold out hope for the promise of health. But the PSA test can also, when used in the diagnostic context of lower urinary tract symptoms, suggest the size of the prostate, because the amount of antigen produced is directly related to how big the prostate is. The bigger the prostate, the more PSA produced, and *vice versa*.

When it is used in this way, the PSA result is compared against the results of the rectal examination and the ultrasound. As a urologist I spoke with said, these three different prostate sizes can be triangulated to give the "true" size of the man's prostate, knowledge that can have significant consequences for further treatment options. And—more specifically related to the PSA results and cancer—if the ultrasound suggests that the prostate is large, whereas the PSA is a little high, then the doctor is less worried about possible prostate cancer than if the PSA is high, but the ultrasound image indicates a small prostate.

Like many of the other tests described in this chapter, the PSA results produce a numerical value that both indicates the number of prostate-specific antigens in a patient's blood and, by reading this value as a result of the prostate size, indicates how big the prostate is. The PSA brackets a whole network of visible and invisible technologies and people, including the patient's blood, his prostate and the prostate-specific antigen, the artifacts used for drawing and analyzing the blood, and laboratory networks to test for the PSA and produce results.[55] Similar to the Qmax score, the PSA produces a number that is used initially to determine the size of the prostate, but also becomes a baseline for the patient to compare future tests against for years to come. The importance of this baseline is not to be underestimated. It is useful for doctors to have for future examinations and to monitor the prostate for potential cancer. And it is used by the patient, who will now become one of the ever-growing group of men who carry a cancer-terror-inspired worry about their PSA numbers for the rest of their lives.[56]

Discussion: Knowing the Prostate

One of the main goals of the rectal examination, the ultrasound examination, and the PSA test is to measure the size of the prostate gland, because this is one of the deciding factors for which treatment method to follow. That said, the size of the prostate is not necessarily an indication of its role in the patient's symptoms. As the European author of a large and thorough treatise on the prostate wrote as early as 1903: "So much is certain, that prostatic hypertrophy is by no means the only cause of bladder insufficiency in old people. There remains a large number of cases which are not accompanied by enlargement of the prostate."[57] The same year one of his North American colleagues, in a collection of survey responses to questions about how to treat men presenting with urinary tract issues, wrote: "The damage being done by an enlarged prostate is by no means determined by its size. The author has very often seen enormous glands that were producing little disturbance, and the other extreme, as well."[58] Medical studies and clinical practice guidelines stress that the connection is tenuous, even today.[59] Attributing urinary issues specifically to the prostate is not a simple matter, even if this is what the medical community started to do in the nineteenth century, and continues to do today.

The most important difference between the examination practices delineated in this chapter is that through the rectal examination, the ultrasound, and the PSA test, the prostate as a thing[60] is known, not the symptoms of LUTS. As opposed to the knowledge created by the symptoms questionnaire, the urination tests, or the medical history, the results of the rectal examination, ultrasound, and PSA examinations create "the prostate" as a stable object. These examinations take as a starting point the assumption that a discrete, bounded prostate exists; it has a size, shape, and consistency, and different methods of knowing it will discover these qualities.

This can be contrasted with the measurements of a man's urination and bother, the first examinations in this chapter, which produce knowledge not about an object, but about experiences. They are measuring practice, often variable over time. They transform a man's urination into a stable, singular number, which allows a variable practice to be stabilized, and can be assigned to and follow the patient through the diagnostic and treatment trajectory. They also transform the patient's subjective complaints about urination into a number that allows comparison between patients and specific pathologies. Like the funnel through which the urine is passed, these diagnostic tests collect the wide messiness of lower urinary tract symptoms, lifestyle practices, and the built environment, and direct them into a single number, a clear and transportable measure.

While the difficulties of knowing the prostate's size are recognized[61] (especially if a transrectal ultrasound is not used), there is still value in investigating the prostate with the rectal examination and the PSA tests. But in this chapter I have discussed how, together with the diagnostic tests that analyze urination, these clinical examinations all bracket the people, infrastructures, and technologies used to produce them, turning the practices of knowing urination and the prostate into facts, numbers, and estimates about the size of the prostate and the patient's lower urinary tract symptoms.

Let me return to the series of questions that were meant to measure how much the patient is bothered by the symptoms, which I discussed at the beginning of this chapter. If we think about this list of questions as a diagnostic technology, it is a tool that both directs the doctor's way of questioning and creates a framework for the patient to use to think about his condition. Through its use in the medical examination, it says something objective about the changed experiences of urination over time. The questionnaire becomes a way of recording this practice, a practice that is usually done in private, away from the prying eyes of doctors or partners. The questionnaire allows the doctor to "see" it. Urination bother becomes stabilized, visible, and transportable.[62] But when the questions are answered and the numerical values are assigned to those answers, those numbers then become lower urinary tract symptoms, possibly even an enlarged prostate, and, later, the success or failure of treatment. The questionnaire's answers initially stabilize the changing values assigned to the practices of urination, but then become, through their shifting roles in the diagnostic and treatment regime, so much more.

With the ultrasound measurements of the prostate, the images created with the probe are granted the agency to articulate "facts" about the size (and to some extent the composition, inasmuch as tumors become visible) of the prostate gland. The same happens with the rectal examination and the PSA. This gland is assumed to exist in a stable form at the time of the examination, even if it is suspected to have grown in the recent past, and will probably continue growing in the future.

The difference between producing a numerical value of an experience and producing a numeral measure of the size of a gland has implications for what diagnosis can be made and where the treatments will be directed. The examinations which create knowledge about the experiences of the patient are making that experience the focus of the diagnosis, and the examinations which create knowledge about the prostate create the prostate as the focus of the diagnosis. These two different foci, the experiences (of urination) and the object (prostate), are combined when they become entangled together into the LUTS/BPH diagnosis.[63]

In chapter 2 I used historical examples to describe a time when the prostate and its health could be a stand-in for talking about appropriate sexuality, masculinity, and vigor. At that time—the end of the 1800s—a man's identity could also be used to discuss and diagnose his prostate, just as his prostate could say something about the man. There may be a tendency to think that medical diagnostic practices are not similarly imbued with overtones of cultural identity today, but the examples in this chapter suggest otherwise. Background questions about the patient's health are meant to give an idea about who that man is and what he has been through before. The "bothersome" questionnaire draws heavily on preconceived ideas about what a man's body should be able to do in various social situations. And the rectal examination is conducted in a way which clearly produces a particular notion of masculinity for the patient.

While it may be surprising to realize how many social practices and norms are bracketed by medical diagnostic techniques for the prostate, this is not necessarily a bad thing. Asking medicine to consider and respect the individual and their social context in diagnostic practices is something patient activism has long agitated for—to get the emotionless, neutral, objective eye of medicine to see and recognize the patient as a person rather than an assemblage of flesh and bones. This way of seeing the body, it could be asserted, would produce knowledge about the prostate-in-the-person[64] rather than the prostate by itself.

The analysis in this chapter has also been inspired by ideas that the material world is created, enacted, and brought into being in very context- and practice-specific ways.[65] How this is done—the details of practice, including the negotiated and taken-for-granted power assumptions and cultural norms bracketed by them—is important for what worlds are enacted and how individuals (and their bodies, organs, and diseases) are allowed to live, are treated, are defined as healthy or sick, given hope or termed chronically ill. As these practices are multiplied, reproduced, spread (for example, through internationally accepted questionnaires, "best practices" policy documents, and clinical guidelines), these ways of bringing into existence people and patients, age, urination practices, and prostates create spaces and definitions within which both "healthy" and "sick" people may be categorized.

Those patients and categories are entangled in diagnostic practices, as detailed here, but they are also affected by their interactions with the physical world we live in. For example, most of us live in a built environment that discourages frequent urination in a public space. But it doesn't have to be that way. One can ask what a public space that allowed for frequent urination would look like. What different facilities would need to be provided? How many more? Where? Our public bathroom infrastructure has changed as a response to social activism in the past, reflecting the entrance of women into the workplace in larger numbers, the civil rights movement, demands for wheelchair-accessible facilities, and trans and nonbinary people's needs.[66] What would a public toilet infrastructure that fits the needs of older men with prostate issues look like? I imagine that it would have receptacles for the disposal of incontinence pads, for one thing. And that it would be more available to those on the move. One can also ask what sort of built environment in the home could be designed to address frequent nocturnal urination? What personal artifacts or interior design changes would facilitate this? Consider the idea that it is widely accepted that one needs reading glasses once one is over forty. One could ask what helpful tools could be used for problems related to an ageing prostate: addressing frequent nocturnal urination, for example, or dribbling.[67] I am not denying that there might be an underlying medical condition affecting changed urination, and this, of course, should be addressed with medical treatments. But those treatments do not have to work in a vacuum. Or would not have to, if we could talk more openly about them. The fact that we do not have these infrastructures or assistive technologies now, or that the need for them is not as commonly spoken about as, say, the need for reading glasses, says a lot about existing taboos and norms. But taboos and norms can be challenged and changed.[68]

Or they can be applied to an ever-widening group. In this chapter I have examined the diagnostic practices of a disease usually found in older men. In the next chapter I will look at a prostate diagnosis that can be applied to younger men, but one which again relies on examinations and treatments that bracket social ways of being to produce the flickering, diseased prostate in an even more foggy and muddled symptom landscape than that for LUTS/BPH.

4

Prostatitis

In chapter 3 I discussed how problems with urination in the older male can become diagnosed as LUTS/BPH, localized to the prostate, and treated as an enlarged prostate. In this chapter, I will be looking at some examples of how diffuse pain in the lower abdomen and urination problems become diagnosed as "prostatitis," even in younger men. Prostatitis is a complex and contested diagnosis, and while I will be writing a bit about the biomedical aspects of it, I will primarily discuss moments in the diagnostic and treatment practices of prostatitis that are specifically related to social masculinities. Additionally, prostatitis, in part because it affects aspects of life related to masculinity, also affects those close to men, especially partners. Prostatitis, like other diseases of the prostate, is thereby a condition which widens its influence beyond the individual body that has been diagnosed with it, to impact on those in relations with that body.

As in much of the rest of this book, the key to under-standing these arguments is trying to open up the conundrum of what prostatitis "is."

Prostatitis presents with a few of the same symptoms as the prostatic hypertrophy of the late 1800s and the LUTS/BPH of today, but not all of them, and often in younger men. However, whereas those first two condi-tions were often associated with an enlarged prostate, prostatitis is not. Rather, prostatitis often presents as diffuse and unspecified pain in the abdominal floor or back. Or—and this is where I begin this analysis—pain and urination difficulties in younger bodies with a pros-tate often become prostatitis.

Even though the research for this book had initially been designed to study the *ageing* prostate, I ended up interviewing younger men as well: men who, for vari-ous reasons, had consulted doctors for prostate prob-lems, and most of whom had been given the diagnosis prostatitis.[1] As one of my informants commented, once he started talking about his prostatitis at parties and at work, it seemed as if every second man he spoke to had had a similar experience, both older and younger men.

Some statistics suggest that half of all men will have a case of prostatitis at some point in their lives;[2] this statistic should be taken with a grain of salt, given that there is no clear definition of what prostatitis *is*. In prin-ciple, the term prostatitis is a collection of syndromes, and attempts to define prostatitis have been made for years. Today there is a general agreement that there are four categories of proper prostatitis: 1. Acute prostatitis; 2. Chronic bacterial prostatitis; 3. Chronic pelvic pain syndrome (which used to be called chronic nonbacterial prostatitis); 4. Asymptomatic inflammatory prostatitis.[3] Patients in categories 1 and possibly 2 have bacterial counts in their semen or prostatic fluid, and can be treated with antibiotics. These are the best-documented categories of prostatitis, but also the rarest. Some people estimate that most (perhaps more than 90 percent) of those with prostatitis are in category 3, the one that nowadays is referred to as chronic pelvic pain syndrome.[4] Chronic pelvic pain is a diagnosis that is gaining ground in Sweden, and even if there are no specialist clinics for this, as there are in England and the USA, there are healthcare centers which are beginning to recruit care providers from different specialist fields who can be engaged around a patient who presents with chronic pelvic pain. But, as noted by one of the coordinators of such a team, it is easy for care providers to miss those presenting with "prostate problems" in their category of patients, as prostate problem patients have traditionally belonged to the urology clinics. The traditional patient group for chronic pelvic pain symptoms more often have a uterus.[5] More on this below.

For those patients presenting with chronic pelvic pain *and* a prostate, doctors tend to try to treat the pain and the prostate with heavy-duty antibiotics. This appears to work in a few cases, but not in the vast majority of patients. Given that bacteria are not found in patients in category 3, antibiotics will do little to relieve the pain, which is why general consensus claims that there is little evidence that antibiotics provide a solution to prostatitis.[6] Overlaid on top of this is a push to prevent the overuse of antibiotics,[7] so many of the men I interviewed in Sweden were not initially prescribed antibiotics in their patient trajectories. And when they eventually were, the antibiotics did not really solve their problems.

For one man I spoke with, the antibiotics he had eventually been given had not worked, and he had instead been encouraged to implement lifestyle changes that would relieve the symptoms. These included watching his liquid intake—he found he could drink no more than one beer in an evening unless he wanted to be up many times during the night—and also making sure he didn't get chilled in the pelvic region. For him, this meant no more fly-fishing. For another man who volunteered his situation to a colleague in this study, it meant wearing long thermal underwear when riding his motorcycle. Staying warm was a common theme.

These examples reminded me of the musings of doctors at the turn of the last century who suggested that being cold and damp, riding horseback in the rain, or some other masculine activity could trigger chronic prostatitis (it was sometimes called this then, as well). As I mentioned above, Björkman and Persson note in their study of the prostate's history that prostatitis was "a catch-all for almost any ailment that a man could suffer from at this time, be it physical, mental, or sexual,"[8] including gonorrhea. However, for the men diagnosed with prostatitis today, gonorrhea is no longer a suspected cause or related problem, as it had been 150 years ago. Looking through the historical material, one sees that when the discovery of antibiotics and their use to cure gonorrhea cleared up this confusion, prostatitis emerged as a problem in and of itself. A letter sent to the *British Medical Journal* in 1948 noted that it was not uncommon for patients to be successfully treated for their gonorrhea, yet still be suffering from prostatitis. These patients were not helped by more antibiotics, nor by massage.[9] Their prostatitis was a curious and muddled condition with a diffuse array of symptoms and an unclear cause. And often it still is today.

While direct associations between sex and prostatitis are rarer now, as late as the 1970s this connection was still being made. Gonorrhea was no longer a suspect, but there were suggestions that perhaps the herpes virus was causing some cases of prostatitis, and that many of the symptoms could be due to lesions on the posterior urethra, or related in some way to sexual function.[10] However, while abstaining from sex and alcohol was recommended in the late 1800s, a century later there was significant doubt about whether abstaining from sexual activity (or alcohol, for that matter) would help those with prostatitis.[11] It was suspected that regular release of the prostatic fluids could be good, and during the 1970s therapeutic prostate massage by a medical professional to produce this fluid release (ejaculation) was considered one line of treatment, though it was generally thought that a series of massage treatments, one or two a week for three to four weeks, would be enough.[12] Today, prostate massage seems to have generally disappeared from the Swedish treatment barrage for prostatitis,[13] though the prostate clinic I visited in 2017 in London employed a clinician who still provided it, and in the US prostate massages are occasionally used to produce fluid for bacterial analysis.

I met several younger men who spoke with me about their prostatitis, but Ali, in his early thirties, epitomized most of the twists and turns of the disease that I also found in the medical literature. I am going to use his experience to explain how prostatitis is understood and treated through both suggested behavioral changes and medicine.

In Ali's case, the progression from pain to prostatitis followed what is probably a pretty common path. He began to feel a specific, localized pain in one of his testicles, but then it disappeared. He thought that maybe he had sat in the wrong position or gotten too cold, but when the pain went away, he stopped thinking about it. Then, though, the pain came back. And then went away again. This continued for quite a while, with the periods of pain lasting anything from a day to a week, but they were always followed by a time without pain that was long enough for him to stop worrying, at least temporarily. After a while the problem began to affect his urination. He began to feel the urge to pee, often quite pressingly, and frequently. When he went to the bathroom and tried to pee, though, nothing happened. At first he had to sit on the toilet for five minutes before he started to urinate. Then it progressed to ten minutes, then fifteen. Nothing would happen, but he would still feel the urge to pee, as if he was about to wet himself. And people started to notice. His partner began to ask what he was doing in the bathroom. At work, he worried that people would wonder why he was always going to the restrooms. And he began to plan his day around his condition, making sure he went to the bathroom at 10.45 if he was going to start a meeting at 11 o'clock. This was about six months after the initial period of pain, and it was the urination problems which triggered his decision to seek medical care:

> "I wanted to be able to avoid worrying about what
> will happen if I can't go to the bathroom when I am
> running from meeting to meeting. That has become an
> extra layer of stress. The physical need to have to go to
> the bathroom and experiencing pain is bothersome. But
> the psychological aspects have been the worst part."

Rather than starting out with the assumption that it might be prostate cancer, Ali first sought help at a sexual health clinic, and ran the gamut of tests for sexually transmitted infections. "Which would have been really odd, since I have had the same partner for a very long time. But I thought I would try that, first." However, those tests all came back negative. Then he tried getting help from his general practitioner, who after three separate visits, including an ultrasound test to rule out cancer, could not find anything wrong either. At the third visit, the doctor was able to localize a pain point in one of the testicles, but nothing more. Yet the general practitioner, following standard procedure in Sweden,[14] was very reluctant to prescribe antibiotics, and instead referred Ali to a urologist for specialist care.

It was at the urology clinic that Ali first received the diagnosis *prostatitis*. He said that within five minutes of meeting the urologist, during which he explained the pain, the urination issues, and the fact that this had all started after an extended vacation abroad which included a lot of swimming in cool water, the urologist was convinced that it was prostatitis, and explained how an infection of the prostate could be related to an infection in the testicle. But he was also very careful to say that there was no guarantee that treatment for prostatitis was going to help. He was clear that this treatment was very difficult, even with antibiotics. And the urologist did not want to prescribe antibiotics right away, either. Instead, Ali was sent back home with instructions to keep warm: wear warmer underwear, sleep with a heated wheat cushion between his legs at night, and take hot baths at least twice a week. If that didn't help, he could come back and they would try some antibiotics.

Two months later, now close to a year after the initial symptoms had appeared, Ali went back to his urologist and got the antibiotics. Even though the urologist was very clear that the antibiotics might not necessarily help, that they made a difference for only about 30 percent of patients, for Ali they did seem to help. Though he did mention that he used them together with the warm baths, the heat cushion, the warm underwear, watching his liquid intake, and a mineral supplement that he had found by Googling. So he was not exactly sure what had helped, but he was inclined to suggest that it was the antibiotics. And he said he didn't feel cured, but he did feel better.

Ali's bouquet of treatments, and the inconclusiveness of antibiotic use, are mirrored in the medical literature. For one thing, not all antibiotics are able to get to the prostate in sufficient concentrations.[15] Other treatments are often suggested, and a recent (2018) Cochrane review compared nonmedical treatments for prostatitis, finding at least some evidence that acupuncture and extracorporeal shockwave therapy (where shockwaves are passed through the skin into the prostate) seemed to have a positive effect,[16] and that possibly lifestyle changes and physical activity might have a (small) effect as well.[17]

In the Cochrane review, prostatic massage also appeared in the list of alternative treatments which had been tested. The reviewers agreed that there was no strong evidence to suggest it had a positive effect,[18] but it is apparently well known enough to become a category of treatment within which one can find studies and results. However, when, during my interview with Ali, I asked if anyone had suggested prostate massage, he just laughed and said: "Only as a joke. Yeah, one of my friends joked about this." But then he went on to reflect over the very idea of a prostate massage, and firmly asserted that it was simply too taboo. "No," he said again, "that could only be the topic of a joke."

It was at this point on his illness path that I met Ali. He was no longer getting up to go to the bathroom four times a night, and his days were not as dominated by the urge to urinate as they had been before. For him, the ratio of discomfort from the body to discomfort from the cure was at a level he could live with. And, significantly, he now knew what was causing the problem: prostatitis. To Ali, just having a diagnosis was a real relief.

> "When I finally got an explanation, it became much easier to handle; just hearing someone say it isn't just in my head. Because I thought for a while that I was going crazy. I was worried that I would be like this for the rest of my life. I was going to be a nutcase and nobody was going to believe me."

Given the examples of connecting the prostate to a man's social and emotional life found in the historical material, Ali's comment did not surprise me. And one does not have to go all the way back to the late 1800s to find examples of how prostatitis is associated with one's state of mind. Depression has lurked in the background as a possible cause much more recently. In the 1970s it was noted that treatment for concurrent depression could sometimes help the symptoms of prostatitis,[19] and by the 1980s, psychological causes for some of the symptoms associated with chronic prostatitis were becoming apparent.[20] Today, mental health issues are still part of the clinical picture, at least in the initial stages of diagnosis.[21] And I have heard urologists discuss men who carry their stress in their pelvic muscles. The idea that there could be a connection between one's state of mind and one's pelvic pain exists today, too.

There is a lively debate about the pros and cons of receiving a diagnosis, but many people, like Ali, feel that getting one and knowing what is wrong is a huge relief. It does, however, also tend to indicate closure of the diagnostic processes, and present a stable disease category. As prostatitis is so complex, and covers so many things, closure may not necessarily be appropriate, and there have been times when doctors have suggested it would be better not to diagnose patients with prostatitis, at least not immediately, because doing so makes it harder to continue discussing other possible causes. As early as the 1980s, doctors were frustrated over the large category of patients diagnosed with prostatitis who did not display any bacterial infections, and there were calls for clinicians to refrain from diagnosing "so-called abacterial" prostatitis without this evidence, so that patients would be willing to continue to search for the true cause of their problems rather than being satisfied with a diagnosis whose treatments would probably not generate a cure.[22] As it is now, large numbers of the prostatitis patient group are being slotted into category 3, chronic pelvic pain syndrome, the group who do not seem to have any bacterial infection and do not respond to antibiotics.

Prostatitis and Urotherapy

During the course of this study, I spoke with a medical professional who was addressing these cases with a different approach. She worked as what is called a *uroterapeut* in Swedish: a subspecialty of medical care that is focused on the pelvic floor region, with particular interest in bladder dysfunction, pelvic floor dysfunction, including difficulties with emptying the bladder, and incontinence. A *uroterapeut* or urotherapist is a medical practitioner who has been licensed after completing a specialty educational program. There does not seem to be an equivalent category in English, though much of what urotherapists do would be at home at a pelvic floor clinic. In Sweden, urotherapists are generally found in adult care clinics, in particular gynecology and obstetrics, but there are connections to urology clinics which deal with bladder problems, as well as to pediatrics, for children with bed-wetting issues.

Most of the urotherapists in Scandinavia are trained nurses who have then become urotherapists, but the urotherapist I interviewed was originally trained as a physiotherapist. At the time of our interview, she was working at the urology clinic of a large hospital; most of her patients were referred to her with functional problems related to urination, as well as pain. Because of this, she treated a lot of patients with prostate problems, both those referred to her by urologists and people who had found their way to her on the Internet and contacted her privately with specific requests to be seen and treated by her. A couple of lectures she has given are online, and these generate quite a bit of interest.[23] "But I have to limit how many patients I take. There are so many, and I'm supposed to do other things, too," she told me.

The prostate patients she meets can have very different types of trouble. Some of them come to her in connection with a prostatectomy which may have caused incontinence; some of them see her because of benign prostate hyperplasia. Some of her prostate patients are referred to her for help with learning how to manage catheters, a technology and technique that she claims is more difficult for younger patients to master than for older ones. And a large part of her patient group are referred to her with prostatitis, which she described as a diagnosis that tends to produce strategies of pain management:

> "Many men with pain in their pelvic region[24] begin their treatments with a urologist. And they get the diagnosis prostatitis. They are almost always treated with antibiotics, often several times, in the hope that

will help. For many of them it doesn't help at all. And
for many with pain, that pain has been there for a
while and it starts to create wider and wider rings in
the water. These men start to avoid situations that
may cause them problems. They find strategies and
work-arounds."

During our conversation, she mentioned some of
those work-arounds: driving a car instead of taking a
bus, so the person is freer to move about and stretch
when necessary to relieve the pain; avoiding certain
foods or drinks; not sitting down for long periods of
time (like Ali, I thought, who mentioned his stand-up
desk as a savior at the office); and avoiding sexual activity if that seems to increase the pain. These are all methods that her patients use to lessen the pain and relieve
the muscle tension in their pelvic region. And they are
all strategies that address and change social aspects of
life that are affected by the development of chronic
pelvic pain. As such, they also involve other people, be
they partners, colleagues, or friends, meaning that the
pain is impacting on a widening circle. Adjusting one's
social activities (transportation, working practices, sex
life) because of pain can have a tendency to isolate the
sufferer from people and activities that are important
to them.

When she and I began discussing this group of
patients, she talked me through the four categories of
prostatitis (mentioned above) and was adamant that
her first concern was to make sure the patient had been

tested for a bacterial infection, and, if that test had been positive, that the patient had actually been given antibiotics. "But," she said, "the majority of prostatitis patients end up in the category of unclear/diffuse trouble with no specific bacterial find. And I think that is because the pain is stemming from something else. And that is why we are using the term CPP, chronic pelvic pain, or CPPS, chronic pelvic pain syndrome." This, she said, was an umbrella term that could be used for patients who presented with pain anywhere in the pelvic region—prostate, sure, but also vulva, or clitoris. The defining features of the pain were that the patient had been experiencing it over a long period of time, that it was chronic, and that it was in the pelvic region. But it did not necessarily need to be located at a specific point—sometimes it could gradually emanate from below the belly, it could hurt when urinating, it could shift focus, or there could be several pain points. But the chronic aspect of it meant that the pain had been experienced for a considerable period of time and that it negatively impacted the individual's quality of life, limiting their ability to do what they wanted to do.

She said that many of her patients were very tense in general, and much of her therapy starts by getting them to loosen up the muscles in the pelvic region. She asks them if there has been an event that initially triggered the pain—perhaps a physical injury, but this trigger could just as easily be a life event: a period of stress, a sexual assault, divorce, or a move.

The urotherapist's focus is very much on the muscles of the pelvic region and their role in pain, but also their role in issues around urination and constipation. She said that during an examination she would ask the patient to take off all their clothes. Then she would examine them for swelling and redness, and ask them to move around the room to see how the muscles of their hips and back worked together. She stressed that pain does not need to occur at the point of damage or stress: that a problem with the knee, for example, could be experienced as pain in the hip. Therefore, she was looking at the patient's body as a collection of interacting muscles. But then, after observing from the outside, her examination practice also included feeling the internal muscles of the lower pelvic region, and this had to be done through an internal, manual examination of the rectum to feel the lower pelvic muscles.

The urotherapist spoke at length about pain; the different ways of treating it, but also the different ways it could appear and inhabit the patient's body. She said how difficult it is to treat long-term, chronic pain, because the patient's body has learned to live with this, to adjust to it, and to expect it. Her words mirrored much of what is happening with chronic pain care and the discussions about how difficult it is to define and treat it. They also mirrored the shift in thinking about pain as a result of a specific cause to thinking about pain as part of a systemic response or psychological state.[25]

Her understanding of pain influenced which treatments this urotherapist suggested to address muscle tensions and possible inflammations of the pelvic area. She could both work with massage to try to loosen up the muscles, but also give the patient a series of exercises to do at home, and sometimes her patients turned to acupuncture and yoga, as well. The purpose of these exercises, and her work with the muscles, was both to create a sense of awareness in the patient of the extreme tension they are holding in their pelvic region, and to create movement in the muscles, relaxing them. At this comment, I started to reflect back on the Cochrane review, and the tension between evidence-based policies and practices (and randomly controlled trials) versus interventions like yoga (or prostate massage) which seem to lack evidence (or perhaps lack the funding for studies that produce evidence) but might just work, anyway. Or might not. How medicine deals with them, in which subspecialties they appear, and how they are articulated or silenced, is constantly changing.

This particular practitioner employed an approach which combined the muscle interests of a physiotherapist with the therapeutic concerns of a urotherapist. However, her background in these two fields is rather unique. One of the difficulties with teaching others to do what she does is that she must either try to get urotherapists with a nursing background interested in the muscles of the pelvic floor, or try to get physiotherapists who are more used to working with other muscle groups to think about the internal muscles of the pelvic floor as a therapeutic location. As she wryly noted, accessing the pelvic floor by a rectal examination is not what physiotherapists are taught to do during their training, and it is not something many of them feel comfortable with. Even though they may be used to examining nearly naked patients in their regular practice, these patients do keep their underwear on. An internal examination of the genital region is potentially embarrassing for both medical practitioner and patient, yet that is what is needed to examine the pelvic floor muscles and start to work on their tensions. As she commented, "The pelvic muscle is the only muscle that we cannot examine from the outside. So I usually show [the patient] pictures of it, and explain that I need to feel it. And many patients are then OK with being examined, because they do want to get help with their pain."

Why Prostatitis?

That prostatitis is a disease of the prostate may seem self-evident from its name, and that is why it is part of this book. But after my interview with the urotherapist, I started to wonder about the connection. There is a strong focus on the *prostate* in the way that the pain is diagnosed as prostatitis. In Sweden, patients—those with prostates—seeking treatment for the pain described above will often be referred to a urologist. Given that urologists are specialists in kidneys, the urinary tract, and the sexual reproductive organs, these are the parts of the patient that will be examined during such a visit. Yet there is still uncertainty about what prostatitis is caused by, and as the Swedish online healthcare advice page says, "It is still unclear why some people get chronic prostatitis. It is seldom caused by bacteria or a virus. Sometimes the prostate is inflamed. But it is common to have pain only in the pelvic floor muscles. It is possible that what today is called chronic prostatitis has completely different explanations for different people."[26] This indicates that prostatitis (like many conditions) is not a stable concept. Its definition is changing over time and across patient groups. It is both "in the making" and, as the shift from "nonbacterial prostatitis" to "chronic pelvic pain" for the third category of prostatitis shows, it is also in the "unmaking." Its ontological status is both multiple and contested. But this status can be articulated through a simple question: Why is the prostate the scapegoat for a condition in which it seems to be neither the site of infection nor the cause of pain in most cases?

In the narratives of the prostatitis patients I interviewed, their pain was in the general region of the pelvis. In this anatomical area, the pelvic muscles share space with the genitals and reproductive organs, including the prostate and the bladder. It would seem logical that one would seek treatment from a doctor who specializes in those organs and that region. For bodies with a prostate, that specialist is a urologist. The same is true for those experiencing difficulties urinating, also a condition that generally ends up in the office of a urologist.

Our specialist medical care structures for the genital and reproductive regions are strictly divided, and categorized by a binary understanding of sex. Bodies with prostates are referred to urologists, a category of experts who do not have the interest or background in pelvic muscles that gynecologists and midwives have because of their involvement with birthing. Pelvic floor muscle therapy is generally considered a useful treatment for pelvises with uteri (and is of particular interest for those pelvic floor muscles that have been involved in pregnancy and childbirth). For patients who have a uterus or have given birth, pelvic floor therapy is often recommended by gynecologists. But if the body experiencing pain in the region has a prostate, and has been referred to a urologist, that discipline's medical toolbox has theoretical knowledge and treatment options more honed to address urination, prostates, pelvic cancers, and erections. Pain and urination issues become prostatitis, which becomes a disease of the prostate and a disease treated by urology rather than, say, physiotherapy, general medication for inflammatory conditions, or psychiatry.

Yet the long-standing and historical anatomical interests of urology are not sufficient to explain why is it that the *prostate* becomes the target of intervention and the source of prostatitis. Most bodies with prostates also have testicles, seminal ducts, a penis . . . different anatomical parts that also belong to the field of urology, and could just as easily have become a point of intervention. Why the prostate? What is being served when the prostate becomes the location of this poorly defined condition with diffuse symptoms?

Perhaps part of the reason can be found in the long shadow of history, and the tendency to draw parallels between the uterus and the prostate in cases of diffuse pain or urination difficulties (see chapter 2).[27] One hundred and twenty years ago, the prostate was being cast in the role of the villain, and remnants of that narrative may remain with us today. Perhaps another clue can be found in the difficulties associated with examining and treating the prostate. The prostate *is* hard to examine. It is stuck inside the body in a place that is hard to reach. It is hard to see. It is hard to touch. You can't smell it, or describe its color; even its shape is tricky to delineate without visualization tools like an ultrasound probe. And it is just as hard to access and know for patients as for doctors. It is a bit mysterious, and as such can easily account for what is, with prostatitis, often diffuse pain and discomfort. It can be an inaccessible, and therewith incontestable, location for that pain, and provide a target for treatment. By localizing the pain and stabilizing its position in the prostate, it also produces a place toward which to direct the treatment.

Getting patients to accept that their pain has a location is not so difficult. More tricky is getting them to let go of that notion: the idea that the pain can be localized to one anatomical place and treated there. This problem is well known and discussed at length in discourses around chronic pain, and was something that the urotherapist brought up during our interview. As mentioned earlier, there is an attempt to stop thinking of pain as something that stems from one source, and instead see it as a systemic response.[28] Using the prostate as a scapegoat for the diffuse and hard-to-define pain of prostatitis would seem counter to the theoretical trends in pain care, but in line with an understanding that patients are wont to accept.

The 2018 Cochrane review I mentioned above is titled "Non-pharmacological interventions for treating chronic prostatitis/chronic pelvic pain syndrome." This title shows how the current understanding of prostatitis is morphing into a definition that includes (and is maybe being slowly challenged by) chronic pelvic pain. It is a discursive shift that can be found in many places, and has been commented upon and generally accepted in the medical literature, even appearing in some online resources.[29] And despite my interviewees' experiences with the diagnosis of prostatitis, it is also a shift that is making its way into diagnostic guidelines and practices. For example, in the current (2020) Swedish healthcare online recommendation pages, chronic prostatitis is equated with chronic pelvic pain. However, one of the glitches in this change is that prostatitis occurs in (adult) bodies with a prostate, but chronic pelvic pain occurs in all bodies, and is in fact probably more widely recognized and more frequently treated in those bodies that do not have a prostate. The trickiness of combining these two names for the syndrome appears clearly in some of the symptoms that chronic prostatitis presents, like shooting pain that spreads to the testicles and penis, or pain during ejaculation. These are symptoms which only a body with a penis or testicles would experience, even though the connection between these occurrences of pain and the prostate gland is not always clear. Yet other symptoms of "prostatitis" are clearly applicable to all bodies experiencing chronic pelvic pain: it hurts when sitting, the sufferer has difficulty or pain when urinating, or feels the urgent need to urinate frequently, often even during the night. All of these symptoms are (also) indicators of the diagnosis for chronic pelvic pain.

When the men I interviewed spoke about their treatment regimes, they did so by recounting their lived experiences of prostatitis. They spoke about how it affected their lives, showing how prostatitis is a physical problem, but one that becomes a social problem because of societal norms, values, and expectations. Take, for example, a doctor's suggestion to avoid getting chilled. That became a problem for the man who enjoyed fly-fishing when visiting his friends and family in northern Sweden, because of its connection to shared social experiences. The same is true of the man who was encouraged to avoid riding his motorcycle unless he wore long underwear. In Scandinavia, some ideals of masculinity (and there are many different ones, of course) are strongly associated with physical activities out in the wild—sailing, hunting, fishing, motorcycling . . . and given the climate, these can involve getting cold. The prostatitis becomes a social problem when it inhibits a man from participating in them.

Similarly, men who spoke to me about consciously reducing their liquid intake in the evening were also adjusting their participation in social contexts that often focused around (alcoholic) liquid intake. In some social situations, being able to "hold one's alcohol" is a socially important skill, and prostatitis impacts on that.

The same sort of analysis can be applied to Ali's comments about his frequent and prolonged visits to the toilet. Yes, the actual urination difficulties were both frustrating and causing worry about the development of the disease. That is very important, and I am *not* saying that prostatitis is only a socially constructed experience of the body. But, at the same time as Ali began to worry about the etiology of the problem, he also worried about what others would think—if his colleagues would notice how frequently he was taking bathroom breaks, if he would be able to sit through a whole meeting without having to go to the bathroom, how to answer his partner's questions about what he was doing in there for so long. These are all social responses from other people to his body's changed practices, and are a result of the fact that he lives with someone else, works in a group, is a social being, just as most men who develop prostatitis are.

This reflection on the social implications of prostatitis and the social production of worry about prostatitis can be useful for two reasons: one, acknowledging it can underline the importance of being able to talk about prostatitis—of lifting it out of silence and brushing away any taboos that might be sticking like cobwebs. By doing so, one could avoid compounding the difficulties of a physiological problem with social complications. In many ways, prostatitis is still silenced. Ali found many men who had experienced it when he himself brought it up at parties. And I have had similar experiences when I have mentioned my research in social settings. But for the most part, men do not seem to be mobilizing around this condition in the same way that patient groups, activists, and celebrities have mobilized around prostate cancer. Why this is would be a topic of another study, though one could start with some of the lessons learned from social science work that has been done on the breast cancer campaigns,[30] or clinical testing on women's bodies,[31] as well as the literature that has examined how women's health activism has become a political force for change.[32] Prostatitis as a diagnosis is not as well-known and generative, nor is it part of a larger movement of men attempting to reclaim their bodies and gain knowledge about them.

But the other, more analytical reason for thinking about the social aspects producing prostatitis is that this, perhaps, gives a clue to why it is still so important for the medical community to employ the term prostatitis even though most patients suffering from it are in the third category, which has been renamed chronic pelvic pain syndrome. Thinking through the social aspects of prostatitis can indicate what work the term prostatitis is doing that chronic pelvic pain cannot. When I was discussing this with my research group, the anthropologist, Gleisner, suggested that it has to do with cultural understandings of masculinity. Imagine being in a situation where you are no longer able to fly-fish in cold water, ride your motorcycle without long underwear, spend a whole evening drinking with the guys . . . or even go to the bathroom when you need to without worrying about what your colleagues or your partner will say, and the suspicious looks they give you as you exit. Now imagine that you had to explain these things with the diagnosis *muscle tension in the pelvic area*—maybe related to stress or lifestyle, a job situation or a divorce—and treat it with yoga, medication, acupuncture, Kegels (aren't those for women???), or pelvic massage. That diagnosis is asking men to trade a prostate issue for chronic pain, a possible infection for a stress response, and motorcycle riding (albeit wearing long underwear) for yoga or meditation.[33] I was immediately reminded of the tendency to feminize men's pathologies that Björkman and Persson found at the turn of the last century. And what man wants to be feminized by a pathology? Keep in mind that throughout this chapter, there have been more bodies affected by the prostatitis than just those that have a prostate. Partners, drinking companions, fishing mates, colleagues . . . these other people have, knowingly or unknowingly, been affected by (and probably had an effect on) the prostatitis. It becomes a disease with cultural contours and, in some ways, labeling this condition as prostatitis produces and reproduces understandings of masculinity held by those around the man as much as by the man himself. That may be important.

But by diagnosing *prostatitis* in those patients who are presenting with chronic pelvic pain and a prostate, we are not only allowing the prostate (a gland of the male body, associated with sexuality and masculinity) to take the blame, we are also claiming that we can treat it and cure the prostatitis. In this way, chronic pelvic pain bodies are still allowed to enact masculinity. This changes the condition to one that reasserts manliness even as it admits a problem, and though the same changes to behavior and social practices may be required, at least it allows these to be made under the banner of a male gland. Since the prostate is also so closely allied with prostate cancer in the *zeitgeist*, the diagnosis additionally allows a sigh of relief. Through prostatitis, one can enact masculinity, *and* at least one does not have cancer.

Does modern, evidence-based medicine take the social, gendered implications of alternative diagnoses into consideration when determining what is wrong with a patient? Of course, the answer is no. But please imagine a very pregnant pause in my narrative right here. Does it? I would never accuse individual doctors of considering what their patient wants to hear before giving a diagnosis that might not fit with the guidelines but may be easier to accept. But that doctor and those guidelines are not working in a vacuum. And as the historical examples I discussed in chapter 2 show, and as the chapter on LUTS/BPH describes, medical diagnoses develop over time, and in response to social understandings and situations. They are entangled with the lived experiences of the embodied subjects to whom they are applied. This has been one of the points of research in the field of men's health and masculinities studies. Men (and not just women) are gendered in particular ways in particular contexts, and this is important to remember when we study how men's bodies and health are medicalized.[34]

I began this chapter with a discussion of what prostatitis is. However, at this point it may be more appropriate to claim that I have really written about what prostatitis is mobilized to do. No one really seems to know what prostatitis is . . . and attempts to pin it down seem to result in multiplicities; definitions that describe variations and symptoms more than actually define a pathology or help a doctor—of any specialization—to diagnose it.

Perhaps this indicates that there are blind spots in our medical knowledge about the male body, a claim that we are more used to hearing in discussions about women's health and female bodies.[35] And, just as academic and activist work within gender studies and feminist theory have helped to address these blind spots in women's healthcare, the same concerns about medicalized bodies (about the individual as an embodied social being, the interplay of norms and values on definitions of health, on expectations of gender and sexuality in relation to bodies and subjects) and the production of medical facts within hierarchies of knowledge (whose knowledge, what research materials, which questions) could also help to articulate the practices, values, and consequences of masculinity for prostate health. Or, perhaps, for pelvic region health. Using lessons learned about, in particular, female reproductive and sexual health, we could start asking questions about prostatitis that probe which silences currently exist, and why we feel more comfortable talking about the prostate than other diffuse pain conditions in the pelvic region. And about why we continue to employ a structure of healthcare provision that reproduces a binary understanding of sex. There may certainly be elements of healthcare that benefit from strict divisions between men's health and women's health. But there may also be diseases and treatments, and patients, that do not benefit from those divisions.

5
The Social Complexity of PSA Screening

"Should I get a PSA test?" During the course of this study, I heard this question a *lot*. Even when it wasn't asked straight out, I could feel it in the air, hovering above my conversations with men about their prostates.

"Is the test any good? How can the PSA number be interpreted? What sort of number *should* I have? What sort of number do I *want* to have? Could I have cancer, or is it a false positive? Do I really need to take the test?" These questions were often asked through a haze of worry—so much so that I started to think of PSA as prostate-specific angst instead of prostate-specific antigen. And that the PSA *test* is causing the angst, not the prostate.

In the first part of this book I examined how knowledge about the prostate—what it is and what it does—is influenced by culturally and historically informed techniques and technologies of knowing the prostate and the patient's experiences of it. Given that the contours of the gland itself are shaped by the cultural prism through which it is viewed, it is not surprising that diseases of the prostate are also affected by social structures and values, which I discussed in chapters 3 and 4. So too, of course, is the PSA test, one of the most lauded yet also most controversial tests for prostate cancer.[1]

But before I get into the complexity of a simple blood test, let me provide a bit of background: prostate-specific antigen (PSA) is a proteolytic enzyme, secreted by the prostate into the ejaculate, that liquefies the seminal plasma, thereby allowing sperm to swim more freely. Small amounts of it also leak into the blood. Measuring this amount in the blood can indicate if there is an increased risk of cancer in the prostate. The PSA test was first experimentally used to detect prostate cancer in the late 1980s, and in the mid-1990s it was approved for this purpose in the USA.[2] However, it is notoriously difficult to interpret, and can be connected to prostate size and age, and to other diseases like BPH, inflammations, and infections (see chapter 3). It can also be prone to false positives. Coupled with the digital rectal examination (feeling the prostate), its reliability can be improved—a bit. It can be used in conjunction with an MRI scan or ultrasound examination to determine prostate volume and tissue structure. Research is currently being done on new methods, like Stockholm3, which would test for aggressive prostate cancer using protein markers, genetic markers, and clinical data.[3] Results of PSA tests can—often do—lead to the next step: biopsy, which is often experienced as unpleasant, sometimes painful, and can lead to blood in the urine and, in some cases, infection. Biopsy following elevated PSA is, however, increasingly being replaced by MRI scans which, no doubt, are less cumbersome and might decrease the risk of unnecessarily detecting small, clinically insignificant, cancers. Nevertheless, results of PSA tests can also—often do—lead to years of repeated, regular testing for the individual patient. And to years of repeated, regular PSA angst. But the PSA test can also lead to the detection of significant, potentially lethal, cancer, and the chance to save a life.

Sometimes, however, the PSA test is the first step to detecting a slow-growing cancer in a much older man. In cases like these, there are those who wonder if detecting the cancer was a good thing, since that cancer might never have caused problems, nor shortened the man's life. If it is detected, the man and his family are placed in the shadow of cancer, faced with decisions about (and, in most countries, costs of) treatments with life-changing side effects. The man and his family are also thrown into a period of worry and anxiety, none of which would have occurred without the PSA test. This is one of the paradoxes of the PSA test: people want it to find cancer and save individual lives, but they also critique it for finding too much cancer and destroying lives when applied across a whole population. For many individual men, even though they know that it might be the beginning of an extended rollercoaster ride of testing and more testing, there is still an almost irresistible impetus to know—and the hope that the test will prove they are—still—cancer-free.

It is this oscillation between hope and fear, combined with the continuous discursive shifting between the PSA as a test for individuals and the PSA as a screening tool for public health at the level of the population, that produces much of the debate about the PSA. In this chapter, I will discuss the complexity of the PSA screening debate and the impossibility of finding one answer to the question of whether it is good to use, or not. I will show how the debate itself gives voice to many different actors—individual men, patient groups, medical professionals and policy-makers—and that each of them has different concerns. And I will point out that this, combined with our fear of vulnerability but inability to fully engage with it within healthcare policy, is why the PSA test, especially as a screening tool, is a cause of so much angst.

Complex, Confusing . . . Collective?

As a critical theorist and medical sociologist, it is its complexity that makes me interested in the PSA test. But even if I hadn't been running this research project, I think I would have been concerned and confused about this test. I hear many of the men around me agonizing over whether they should take it, wondering how they should interpret the results, and, most troublingly, intensely worrying about possibly having cancer in the weeks leading up to their test appointment, and in the intervening time between leaving the blood sample and getting the results. Men whom I otherwise think of as healthy, busy, engaged in work and social activities become, in the face of a blood test, worried and preoccupied with their mortality.

This preoccupation is not uniquely related to the PSA test—we are, after all, mortal. And especially at a certain age, most of us start to reflect upon this. However, the angst I see these men experiencing seems specifically generated by the threat of prostate cancer that the PSA test causes. Of course, that threat is biologically always present, and we should be aware of what the prominent position of prostate cancer in the general *zeitgeist* does to men of a certain age (of many ages, really). But there is something special about the PSA test. It is a test that congeals that angst into a worry which eats away at many men.

When I am having these conversations—with friends, with colleagues, and with men I have interviewed—I tend to remember a urologist I met early on in this study, who admitted slyly that he didn't get the PSA test for himself, to avoid, as he called it, "starting down that slippery slope." He wasn't the only urologist who admitted this to me during the course of my study, and his comment articulated a well-known phenomenon: that testing and screening can lead to a series of further tests, and a future of uncertainty. And sometimes it can generate pre-illness, proto-illness, or the idea of being a patient-in-waiting;[4] even if you are not sick now, testing and screening can produce the feeling that you might become sick, that you might develop symptoms, and that in the future you will be struck by, in this case, prostate cancer.[5] Then, once you have been tested, you as a patient are responsible for getting tested again, and keeping track of your numbers, following their ups (ideally not) or downs, or just their steady onward march through time. The numbers[6] become a visible way of knowing what is happening in your body, of trying to pin down risk and uncertainty.[7] But because the PSA test can also be the first step in a series of more invasive tests, including biopsies, scans, and, if needed, surgical or other procedures to treat cancer, it is also cracking open the door to a future that threatens the side effects of prostate treatments, like impotence and incontinence and the feelings those possibilities evoke. It raises the specter of cancer and death. Medical experts and policy-makers are aware that PSA testing is a source of anxiety for patients, but there is scant research on this,[8] and what little there is tends to be mentioned but not considered seriously in debates about screening and testing decisions. This seems particularly poignant in recommendations that, more recently, have encouraged patient participation in deciding whether to test or not,[9] a situation in which anxiety over results and potential false positives conflicts with the anxiety about refusing available medical tests and thereby missing a cancer.

This is amplified by the fact that the PSA test is purported to save lives by identifying tumors early, allowing for more successful treatments of smaller, contained cancerous tumors, and ultimately helping to reduce the number of men who die of prostate cancer every year. Public discussions about the PSA test are filled with survival stories from men who have found their cancer (often early, often when they were young) and been successfully treated, so that they are alive today because of it. In these narratives, early detection is considered a good thing, because one is still alive; discussions of side effects are minimal. The PSA test allows medicine to come in and save a life rather than watching impotently by the patient's side through the advanced stages of cancer.

Survival rates for prostate cancer *have* improved significantly over the last thirty years, but it is not clear if this is because of better treatment and primary care, or because of wider screening practices that allow earlier detection,[10] or a combination of both. And while there is agreement that screening could save lives by detecting and treating prostate cancer earlier, it appears to entail the overtreatment of large numbers of men. This means that many men are unnecessarily subjected to surgery or radiation, and thereby have to deal with the severe side effects of treatment: pain, incontinence, bleeding, fistula formation, bowel trouble, sexual dysfunction, etc., as well as the status of patient (including repeated PSA tests post-treatment to monitor if the cancer returns) for years to come.[11] And while the medical community is generally in agreement that many prostate cancers do not need to be treated (especially in men over seventy-five), while others can benefit from active surveillance instead of immediate treatment,[12] it can sometimes be hard to convince a patient of that. Cancer is terrifying. A patient who finds out they have cancer wants to get rid of it, and as quickly as possible. The concept of watchful waiting or active surveillance, however medically justified it might be, could quickly become an emotional nightmare.

The controversy about screening has become entrenched as many national healthcare policy-makers have suggested that men should *not* be screened for prostate cancer with the PSA test. Pushing back against these decisions are national and international patient activism campaigns that try to raise awareness of the importance of screening, and encourage men to get tested. Social responses to medicine have often relied on the strength of collectives rallying around a single health issue: for example, HIV/AIDS or breast cancer.[13] These collectives rely on the political traction a unified voice can exert. This is also true of a particularly male disease like prostate cancer, and there are very vocal collectives forming around it,[14] using arguments about the equitable provision of healthcare for men and the need for special emotional support to deal with the impact of prostate cancer on masculinity and sexuality, parallel to what one can see with women's health issues. In these discourses online, in advertising campaigns, in media reports, etc., anxiety and illness are used in particular ways in relation to masculinity and prostate cancer, including by—but not limited to—prostate support groups.[15] The importance of being tested—and possibly of screening populations of men—is a popular cause for many national prostate cancer patient groups (like Europa UOMO; the French Association Nationale de Malades du Cancer de la Prostate; the German Bundesverband Prostatakrebs Selbsthilfe; the international Movember Foundation; the Swedish Prostatacancerförbundet), even if some countries' patient groups are more reticent (like British Prostate Cancer UK), and even as the medical debate about its validity is still ongoing.[16] Collectively, there are groups of men (and women, and cancer industry interests) promoting PSA and prostate cancer screening and testing, collecting research money for technological development, lobbying for screening programs,[17] and enrolling men to participate in support groups and patient activism. And encouraging men to get tested.[18]

All these voices, interests, and opinions are debating, promoting, rejecting, and encouraging the PSA test as a screening tool in the media around us. Especially in November. November—or Movember—has been the internationally successful flagship promotion campaign of a prostate cancer charity, encouraging men to get their PSA tested and asking them to take individual responsibility for the test rather than relying on national screening policies. This is the message behind the mustache campaigns in November, for example, often fronted by famous men and women with mustaches, that pop up in media outlets each winter. Some years, Movember and the mustaches seem to be everywhere. But notice the shifts I have made in this section: from talking about individual men and their feelings about a simple PSA test to a discussion about the statistical life-saving it might achieve, to the response of governments and professional associations, to patient groups and charities who return the question to individual men and ways of encouraging them to be tested. The shifts from individuals to collectives and back to individuals in the debate can make one dizzy. It is no surprise that people become confused about the value of the PSA test, and its benefit to men.

Sweden's Recommendations against Screening

I sometimes feel, however, that the complexity of the discussions gets oversimplified in public debate. Just such a debate flared up in Sweden in 2018, when the National Board of Health and Welfare decided (again, prolonging a similar decision from 2014) not to suggest a nationwide screening program for prostate cancer using the PSA test.

The Swedish National Board of Health and Welfare had based their decision on the conclusion that the benefits of PSA screening would not outweigh the negative effects for men who were treated unnecessarily, though it did leave open the possibility that developments in other testing technologies that could be used as a complement to the PSA test might eventually change this equation. This decision was immediately met with criticism from some urologists and prostate cancer patient groups, the latter of which also mobilized a media campaign engaging well-known Swedish men in support of PSA testing. The campaign brought forward arguments about early detection, saved lives, and equitable healthcare provision. It was suggested that since Swedish women were called to regular mammograms for breast cancer screening,[19] denying men nationwide PSA screening meant that men were being deprived of equal healthcare. (Swedish women are also called to regular pap smears to detect cervical cancer, but that screening was not mobilized discursively to the same extent, perhaps reflecting the taboo on genital cancers and the saturation of breast cancer awareness.)[20]

This PSA screening decision was in line with Swedish healthcare policy over the previous twenty years. While different voices have promoted the development of PSA screening programs for the early detection and treatment of prostate cancer, regulatory boards and health authorities in North America and Western Europe have not received such recommendations with enthusiasm, citing large-scale studies which question its benefits,[21] an ambivalence found in other parts of the world, too.[22] Additionally, there is legitimate medical concern that the test is not robust enough, that "healthy" PSA levels can vary across populations, ethnic groups, and geographical regions,[23] and that our current understanding of what a healthy PSA level is has been based largely on populations of white men.[24] (Access to and use of PSA tests also varies across ethnic groups, especially in the USA, as does access to care for and mortality from prostate cancer.)[25] Because of this, calculations based on PSA scores are constantly being debated and fine-tuned in order to interpret the results better.[26]

These policy decisions show how international technologies of prostate cancer screening refract local norms about healthcare provision in different nation-state contexts, including their structures around access to healthcare and trust in experts and authority.[27] Thus, at the nation-state level around the world, the question of whether to provide prostate cancer screening has become an issue that healthcare policy-making bodies are still dealing with today, even as most are recommending against general PSA screening and in favor of patient collaboration in testing choices,[28] or providing alternative screening options rather than the PSA, as in Germany.[29] Other countries are just now considering the option of providing the PSA to their populations or encouraging men to seek out the test themselves (sometimes after high-profile prostate cancer cases, as with the former president of Colombia), while other nations are revisiting decisions to not screen in light of new screening technologies and in response to concerted campaigns from patient organizations, as in Sweden.[30] At the same time, in some countries, like Singapore, there is little public debate about the decision not to offer screening.

I started this section with the assertion that in 2018 the Swedish National Board of Health and Welfare decided not to support nationwide population-based screening (which could have taken the form of, for example, sending a letter to every man at the age of sixty offering him an appointment for a PSA test). While this is true, the National Board of Health and Welfare is an organization which offers official *suggestions* for healthcare policy. The *actual* healthcare policies are put into action by the various regional councils in the different counties of Sweden. A nationwide guideline by the National Board of Health and Welfare is not a law or even a practice decision, but only a guideline, a suggestion. Usually the suggestions made by the Board *are* put into practice, but in the case of the PSA examination, some regions did not comply. The most southerly region of Sweden, for example, decided to offer PSA "tests" to all men between the ages of fifty and seventy.[31] While they called this a test rather than a screening, it was to be offered in a letter, sent to each man's home, on the basis of his age and regardless of his individual risk as calculated through earlier diagnosis or a family history of prostate cancer. It was a policy decision that simultaneously challenged the national policy guideline and pointed to a tension in the definition of what is a "screening" policy and what is a "testing" policy.

This discursive conflation of screening and testing is not uncomplicated. Nor is it particularly unusual.[32] Diagnostic testing becomes screening when the target shifts from an individual to a population. Or in this case, screening becomes testing, because the target officially shifted from a population to an individual—but many individuals, in one geographic region, within a particular age span. You can see where this is going. It is still, kind of, screening. Definitions of and criteria for screening are produced by national and international bodies,[33] and it is not uncommon that much of the ethical debate about screening is framed in broad terms of cost–benefit analyses[34] and the relative usefulness (or not) of reducing the burden of disease for a population.[35] But it can also be framed in terms of the individual's right to know, or the possibility for the individual and their families to prepare for potential disease, thus shifting the subject of the debate from the large group or population to the individual or family unit. Sometimes, though not as frequently, the negative implications and consequences for individuals of screening are discussed,[36] but these nuances about what screening is, whom it targets, and what (else) it is doing are often more present in theoretical, academic discussions found in medical ethics debates than in media coverage.[37] At least in Sweden, but I suspect in other places, too. These discussions need a slow and steady pace, and the word counts, column inches, or prolonged scrolling that most media channels do not provide.

Bringing the Discussion into the Living Room

In 2018, the PSA screening debate played itself out in the Swedish national print and TV media as well as in social media bubbles, with their tendencies toward loud and quick exchanges and heated replies. But none of these formats really lent themselves well to in-depth discussions, nor did they necessarily allow different voices and perspectives to come to the table and carefully explain their point of view. To try to facilitate such a discussion, some colleagues and I arranged a scientific salon to discuss the details of PSA screening in Sweden. This may have been mildly pretentious, with a format inspired by eighteenth-century salons, but its goal was to gather together participants who do not normally have the time or place to engage with each other conversationally, and who come from very different facets of the debate. We wanted to provide the chance for them to speak, listen, and discuss, in a relaxed environment, over a bit of food and wine. The conversation was then to be summarized and published online,[38] to take the concerns raised that evening outside of the closed room and into the public domain, but without the demand for argument, catchy sound bites, and headlines.

We held the salon on what turned out to be a cold winter evening, on the top floor of an old palace built in the 1500s, in the center of Stockholm. We placed it there so that we could be close to the parliament building, because we wanted to invite politicians who decide on many of the structures that shape Swedish healthcare. We also wanted to be close to the Stockholm-based workplaces of many other decision-makers and interest groups. We needed the salon to be easy to get to *and* evocative enough to tempt decision-makers out on such an uninviting evening.

I don't live or work anywhere close to penthouse apartments in the medieval city center of Stockholm, so I took the train into town that afternoon. As I was walking from the station, the cobblestones were slippery from the drizzle that had kept the city in a gray cloud all day, but now that the sun had truly set (though, honestly, it barely seems to rise in Sweden at that time of year) the golden light from the antique street lamps and Christmas decorations, and from the cafés and restaurants that line the narrow streets in the old city, all reflected warmly off the wet stone surfaces. Just approaching the salon seemed to calm one down and produce a mindset of reflection. And, I hoped, set the mood for civil conversation.

The host of the salon, in addition to having been a well-known cardiologist, had held several different important decision-making positions in Swedish medical policy and practice during her career. Her participation was a calculated draw, and it worked. Thirty-five people gathered that evening, including politicians, science journalists, practicing urologists, other medical professionals, policy-makers, and patient group representatives, many of whom were prostate cancer survivors themselves. We all found seats in the bohemian furniture of the large living-room and tried to make small talk over a glass of wine and roasted nuts before the event started.

To open the conversation, we had invited three speakers: a professor of urology at the main research hospital in Sweden; a medical humanities professor conducting research into the lived experiences of medical screening; and the chairman of the Swedish National Council on Medical Ethics, the official body tasked with evaluating medical ethics questions in Sweden. Each was asked to specifically address PSA screening from their perspective for ten minutes, before we opened the floor to questions and comments. When we first introduced them, we also asked the others in the room to introduce themselves, so that everyone knew who was there, and we could have a more open conversation after the speakers' talks.

The urology professor began by giving many of the medical facts I have discussed already in this chapter. He talked about how the PSA test was problematic and how it carried very specific risks with it, including further testing and biopsies, increased patient anxiety, and the current uneven access to the PSA test throughout Sweden. This last aspect is a significant problem in Sweden, a country dedicated to providing equal access to equal care for everyone. His talk also touched on how the debate about PSA screening is complicated by technological attempts to improve it.

The medical humanities professor then put medical screening in a larger, social perspective and provoked questions about what patient subjectivities were created by screening, and what it feels like to be an individual called to a test who suddenly becomes a *potential* patient with *potential* pathologies. Her presentation touched on the consequences of screening for both individuals and society, but she also spoke to the way people are informed about the screening opportunity. She questioned the ability of individuals to actually say "no" to the offer of a PSA test when that offer is made from the imagined monolithic fortress of expertise that evidence-based medical knowledge can seem to be. And she spoke about the way a PSA result can be relayed to the individual, calling for more thought to be put into the phrasing and language used in letters and conversations: into the practices of communicating with patients.

The third guest, the medical ethicist and a former medical professor himself, discussed the three central principles that the Swedish ethics board attends to in their decisions about medical care: the human dignity principle, the needs and solidarity principle, and the cost-effectiveness principle. Additionally, he reminded the room, the ethics board must base their decisions on scientific facts. This speaker pointed out that unorganized screening, sometimes called opportunistic screening, when patients or care providers decide to initiate testing on a case-by-case basis, can also lead to inequitable access to care, and to inefficiency. And he pointed out, again, that while lives may be saved by screening, it would also lead to a much larger group of men being unnecessarily diagnosed with, and even treated for, prostate cancer, and perhaps experiencing severe side effects as a result of that treatment.

After their presentations, the rest of the room was invited to ask questions or come with comments to the speakers. The representative from a local prostate cancer survivor group emphasized the importance his organization and the individual men he represented put on the availability of PSA screening. He underlined their disappointment with the decision not to offer nationwide, population-based screening in Sweden. One of the urologists in the room emphasized the PSA test's role as only one tool in a wider spectrum of testing technologies and techniques to detect prostate cancer. And the evening's most interesting comment came toward the end of the session, when a politician from southern Sweden addressed the medical humanities professor with a specific question about patient information sheets—those information letters that are sent to men's homes in conjunction with the opportunity to take a PSA test.

The politician who asked the question about patient information sheets was from that region in southern Sweden I mentioned above. Her question, triggered by the professor's discussion of the emotional impact of screening/testing, was, simply: "You say that the mere act of being offered a testing opportunity can trigger difficult and uncomfortable thoughts about a man's mortality. You say that we should both be aware of this impact of screening opportunities ourselves, and make the man we are sending the information to aware of it, as well. But how do you formulate a brief and simple sentence about that in a one-page information sheet? How can we carefully and concisely warn the person that the act of testing/screening might trigger difficult thoughts about their own death?" Especially, one could add, when merely receiving such a letter in the post may do that.

This question mirrored exactly what the professor had been trying to express. Screening is an option for prostate cancer, as detailed here, and for other pathologies, like breast cancer, cervical cancer, colon cancer, and dementia. But in all of these cases, it does much more than just identify a disease, early signs of a disease, or a risk of developing a disease. It also produces a patient subjectivity for the body being tested.[39] While the diagnostic tools for testing often employ the same technology as the diagnostic tools for screening, the contingencies of their use on an individual body that is displaying symptoms, or on a population of potentially healthy bodies, are very different. And yet we have to remember that populations are collections of individuals. The medical humanities professor was suggesting that screening decisions at the population level should also consider the affective responses to testing for the individual. It is necessary to include an individual's experience of PSA anxiety, anxiety about living with a new identity and possibly a diseased body, in the screening debate.

But with her question, the politician also put her finger on a very sensitive spot in healthcare provision: healthcare as we know it today is governed in this way—with information sheets and short, simple sentences that simplify and flatten complexity in an attempt to achieve clarity. Often, this does away with complexity altogether.[40] The politician's question took for granted the form of governance that we have: one which does not always work, and definitely does not allow for the nuances of a debate like the one engendered by PSA screening.

Her question also opened up a discussion about how we should broach the topic of death, fear, and vulnerability. A lot of healthcare practice and policy is uncomfortable with recognizing death, fear, and vulnerability. And not just healthcare providers and policy makers: also people, us, everyone we know—the users and patients of modern healthcare are uncomfortable around recognizing death, fear, and vulnerability.

I was reminded of this when I was putting forward a draft of this chapter to my department seminar. I had emailed it out to a few different mailing lists, asking people to read and comment on it. Just before the seminar, an older colleague called me into his office. He had read it, and had some very useful comments to give me. But he also felt very uncomfortable attending the seminar because his comments would have outed him as "that guy with a prostate problem." He did not want his professional identity connected to that vulnerable identity.

I was very grateful for his comments, and for his reflections on the way making them made him feel. And that he could articulate how strongly his experiences of the PSA test resonated with the uncomfortable complexity that the PSA test produces.

The existence of the PSA test implicitly produces an individual's responsibility to be tested: to take *individual* responsibility for one's vulnerability to cancer. But that individualization of vulnerability does something more. It produces an individual patient from a social subject, and can, perhaps because of the stigma attached to prostate cancer and treatment side effects, isolate that subject, distancing him from social relations that could have been able to mitigate, or at least placate, vulnerability. Another colleague of mine, Maldonado Castañeda, has compared the PSA test with the pap smear for cervical cancer.[41] His work illustrates the difficult patient–subject position that these tests create for individuals. He has asked how prostate diseases and health can be thought of within wider relations and social constellations, rather than being presented as an individual responsibility with a moral imperative to maintain health through regimes of testing.[42] As he wrote in his analysis of PSA tests: "Vulnerability is a relational state. It is linked to the precariousness of being embodied subjects—being a body—but also to relationships of care and dependence with other people, significant others, family, friends, colleagues, fellow citizens, the government, and the world. Situations of illness and disability are an essential part of the human living experience. They transform us, re-creating social relations of care and dependence."[43] The PSA test—especially when it is offered to individuals, but also when it is promoted as a screening technology—produces vulnerable individuals, then does not talk about that vulnerability, even as it transforms and potentially isolates that individual.

This is why—returning to the salon—I was so glad to hear that question of how to address this raised by the politician. The question indicated and enacted recognition of how vulnerability is produced—not just by life, but by medical practices as well—and made space for a responsibility to acknowledge and mitigate that.

There is no easy answer to the politician's question. How do you take something complex and make it simple, while maintaining the complexity? And how do you warn about the completely rational and expected worry about death that testing might trigger? I won't pretend that the room came up with an answer that evening, because we didn't. That is a very complicated issue. But even though no good answer was put forward, the people at the salon were being forced to formulate the question for themselves and the whole room. We were all made to think through the consequences of testing/ screening decisions beyond the (also very complex) discussions of what is medically advisable. The room was asked to ponder what other consequences the screening might have for those being enrolled into a medical system by the simple, ostensibly generous, offer of a doctor's appointment. No one wants to die of cancer. But a simple blood test to find the amount of prostate-specific antigen in a person's blood does much more than detect a possible prostate cancer tumor, and potentially save a life, no matter how good or how bad that test might be. The salon managed to open up a discussion about some of the other things that might impact on the use and reception of PSA screening.

What to Do with Complexity—or How Not to Make It Simple

The question of PSA screening and PSA testing is more complicated than merely a question of whether the test is good enough or not. It is not only about the risk of false positives—though it *is* about that. It is not only about the risk of overtreatment—though it is about *that*, too. It is not only about the impossibility of screening men, finding cancer, and then being able to know which cancers are dangerous enough to warrant treatment and which are harmless enough to not bother about or embark upon active surveillance. And it is not only about the impossibility of reassuring someone with cancer that they can continue living with it, that they shouldn't worry. It is about all of these things, entangled together.

The conversation that night at the scientific salon did not determine whether or not the PSA test should be implemented as a population-wide screening. We did not come to a conclusion about whether or not an individual should go to their doctor and demand a PSA test, or find a specialist who will provide it if their regular doctor says no. Rather, the conversations that night, and the many scientific studies referenced in this chapter, show that the PSA test involves many voices, perspectives, concerns, and stances. And there is no closure to the debates about its usefulness, even when there is a policy decision. This is because the medical evidence, should it ever become clear, is only one part of the answer.

Judging by the conversation at the salon, the discussions I've had with men during the writing of this chapter, and the voices raised for and against PSA screening in the media, it would seem as if our responses within this regime of anticipation are (at least also) colored by strong feelings of fear and worry about our mortality and vulnerability. A state of affect is not necessarily the most productive place in which to make a rational, calculated decision. And we are often caught in these knots of emotion, statistical risks, and prevention discourses, aided and abetted by well-meaning health promotion campaigns and evidence-based anticipation regimes, a situation that can easily become affective and infected.[44]

We assume that we are rational, calculating agents, making decisions based on objective facts, and we would like to believe that the answers to our screening questions could be based only on objective medical knowledge, because that would suggest that there should be a correct answer out there to questions of screen or test, when and how. But as the very idea of pure medical facts becomes tainted by the undercurrent of social context within which they are being produced, that option fades away. Those decisions about screening that we are living with today are historically formed and culturally embedded, and will always be so. They will engage our feelings of fear and worry specifically because they address mortality and death. This is the unavoidable "affective." But instead of seeing that as a starting point for an infected debate, I suggest we embrace it. Perhaps recognizing those feelings and other social considerations in our decision-making will produce more humane, and ultimately more caring, policies for those we are trying to help.

6
The Absent Prostate

The original title of this research project was "A Constant Torment: Tracing the Discursive Contours of the Ageing Prostate." As I said in chapter 1, I thought we would be focusing only on ways that older prostates were causing problems in the body: on how they were discussed in medical literature and in the cultural imaginary as enlarged, infected, or cancerous, for example. But it soon became clear that not only would we be dealing with discussions about the prostate in younger men (see chapter 4), we would also be confronted by the *absent* prostate, the prostate that has been surgically removed, scraped away from the inside, radiated, electrocuted, microwaved, pharmacologically shrunk, or otherwise destroyed. The missing prostate was the discursive—and very real—source of at least as much torment as a still-present-in-the-body prostate.

This absent prostate appeared everywhere: in medical literature, pop-cultural texts, media debates, and the interviews my colleagues and I conducted. The absent prostate was, at least sometimes, even more present than it had been before it was removed or destroyed. A healthy prostate just sits quietly in the body, doing what it is supposed to do. A diseased prostate starts to cause symptoms, often pain and voiding problems for the body. But an absent prostate, and the damage from whatever treatments it has been subjected to, can produce side effects that remind the person of its (prior, now missing) presence every day.[1] In many of the discourses we examined, the ill-boding duo of incontinence and impotence made up the new and very prominent contours of the prostate.

As you may remember, in chapter 2 I looked at historical explanations of voiding issues and prostate problems, many of which fell back on explanations based on a man's behavior and its relationship to his health. The prostate was associated with masculine physical activities, like horse-riding in the damp and cold, or long hours of office work. The historical material also contained elements of sexual morality, blaming prostate problems on sowing wild oats in one's youth, or marrying a younger wife in the autumn of one's life. These connections were complicated by the prostate's uncertain conflation with long-term, low-grade gonorrhea. Treating the prostate was thought to be important for society at large 120 years ago, not least because of its relationship to hegemonic masculinities as performed in sexual relations, the family, and industry.

In chapters 3 and 4 I discussed traces of social understandings of masculinity in modern prostate discourses—

physically demanding sports, outdoor activities like golf, and road trips are used in pharmaceutical advertisements for prostate medications, for example. Normative understandings of urination are based on and impact on how our public events and spaces are organized: everything from seventh-inning stretches at baseball games, standard movie lengths, and golf courses, to the building regulations for designing public toilets in stadiums, cinemas, and city centers. These examples show, if not parallels between the nineteenth-century understandings and current, modern discussions of the prostate, at least similar mechanisms which now associate the (healthy) prostate with productive masculinity in the workplace (being able to sit for long periods versus having a stand-up desk, being able to attend long meetings, using the bathroom quickly enough), and with participating in masculine leisure activities like motorcycle-riding without long underwear or fly-fishing in cold water.

All of these activities can potentially be affected by the side effects of removing a prostate. Yes, probably the most commonly talked about side effect of prostate treatments is erectile dysfunction, and I'll get to that soon. However, worries about voiding urgency, incontinence (of both sorts), and strategies for dealing with changed urination patterns also appeared everywhere as I conducted this research. When impotence and incontinence are combined, and then mixed with the experience of having a life-threatening disease, the period after prostate cancer treatment can be very challenging for men, physically, emotionally, and psychosocially.[2] I will now discuss the challenges of incontinence, impotence, and the angst of the absent prostate.

Incontinence

The impact of prostate-treatment-related urinary incontinence is, for many people, large and difficult. Many of the men I spoke with talked about how their prostate problems had changed their way of being in the public sphere. Knowledge about this is nothing new; longitudinal studies like the Olmsted one (see chapter 3) have looked at how prostate issues affect behavior like going to movies, taking long car trips, and outdoor sports. As I mentioned earlier, that the body makes itself known through our ways of being in the world is a standard assertion in medical humanities studies, especially the way the body makes itself loudly, painfully, and incessantly known when it is diseased, while the healthy body is a silent body.[3] Incontinence makes the body known. Surgical procedures have been developed to treat it, and an industry producing incontinence pads exists to provide for it. Many men first find they need large pads—and pejoratively take to calling them diapers—but with time, most men can begin to use smaller incontinence pads. Commercial market forces have responded to this need, producing pads in dark, masculine packaging to differentiate them from feminine products. There *are* solutions and work-arounds to urinary incontinence, but it still impacts on a man's life, often seriously.

However, the surprising thing that emerged from my interviews was the awareness of how a post-prostatectomy man's body was *suddenly* not a good fit for the public toilet infrastructure of the built environment *any more*. This changed awareness of an infrastructure that had previously been so well suited to their needs that they hadn't thought about it caught many of the men I met off-guard. In interviews (and informal after-dinner conversations at parties) I would hear about how a man now suddenly knew where the most convenient public toilets were, or which bus rides would be OK and which would be too long, given their leakage or their voiding urgency issues. It was as if their bodies were no longer the imagined standard body for which the public toilet infrastructure was made. Actually, their bodies *were* no longer the imagined standard body for which the public toilet infrastructure was made. That sudden awareness made what had previously been a transparent infrastructure painfully visible.[4] In many ways, it reminded me of the situation I was in when I was pregnant or, later, in town with a small child who was potty-training. Suddenly my needs for a public toilet were different from the imagined needs for which whoever designed the infrastructure had planned. I had always assumed that the public toilet infrastructure had been designed for men, and that was why it didn't fit my needs in these cases. What I came to see in the course of this research is that it had been designed for *some* men (younger, cis male able-bodied ones with healthy, untreated prostates) and that just as feminist research has argued for a heterogeneous, intersectional understanding of the category "women," so too must we employ a nuanced, intersectional understanding of the category "men." This applies to academic writings, but also when one is irritably mumbling under one's breath about the lack of clean toilets in public spaces.

When I brought up this reflection during an interview with a psychologist at the men's health clinic, he pointed out that changed urination patterns can come as a cold shower for many men after prostate treatments—they suddenly realize that they have to adjust their lives to a new body and new bodily needs. He also said that responding to this can either take the form of finding coping mechanisms, like downloading an app that shows where the best toilets are, or always carrying a little change for the pay toilets in town. Or it can prompt avoidance behavior.

Take, for example, going to the theater. Perhaps a man who had always enjoyed going to the theater will, after a prostatectomy or upon the development of prostate issues, stop going out at all because he doesn't want to worry about what would happen if he had to go to the bathroom during the show. Or, worse yet, worry that he wouldn't be able to control his bladder on the way to the restroom. Perhaps he starts to sit at the end of a row, on the very edge of his seat, despite the column that blocks part of his view. It can happen even though the man has possibly never been in the actual situation where he had to go to the bathroom urgently during a show. The mere anxiety about it happening is enough to change his behavior.

This psychologist could see the avoidance behavior extend to other parts of life, too. Perhaps the man will stop taking long-haul flights, even to visit close family, because he is worried about accessing and using the small, often busy, toilets on the airplane. Or stop visiting loved ones, or any other activity which he is no longer willing to try, but which had been something he enjoyed, something that helped him feel good about life. Avoidance responses to incontinence or other voiding issues can lead to isolation, loneliness, and depression (as can prostatitis; see chapter 4). This particular psychologist tended to focus on finding solutions around the problem, to develop coping strategies. When he worked with men, he was meeting them one on one, helping them as individuals. But we could also respond to this worry collectively, changing the infrastructure and developing technical solutions like the public restroom apps or more frequent facilities in the public space.[5] Both a better infrastructure and successful individual coping strategies may be necessary, if we don't want to let men with voiding problems silently drift into the background and stop doing the things they had enjoyed before they developed prostate cancer.

Impotence

Perhaps the most feared side effect of prostate treatments (mostly prostate cancer treatments) is that a man will become, at least for a time, impotent.[6] He will lose his ability to have an erection, which can be very difficult for many men to deal with. With recovery, the erection might come back, but it might be softer than it used to be. Erectile dysfunction is not the only sexual side effect of treatment that may appear, either. Perhaps the man will no longer ejaculate at orgasm, and ejaculate has been an important part of his sexual practice.[7] Or perhaps urine will leak out, instead. There can be other changes, too. Perhaps he will experience pain during sex—at orgasm, for example—or maybe the experience of prostate or anal stimulation will be affected—either lessened or perhaps even painful, at least initially. Maybe his desire will decrease, especially in cases where hormone therapies are involved. Or his sexual satisfaction. There is a plethora of side effects to consider, yet in many cultural imaginaries of prostate treatment side effects, it is erectile dysfunction that looms large. Attached to this fear, seemingly almost inevitably, are often found both heteronormative presumptions[8] and emotional associations with failed masculinity.[9]

The sexologist who worked with our team, Danemalm Jägervall, writes about the complexity of providing rehabilitation for men who have undergone prostate cancer treatments.[10] She is employed at a urology clinic in southern Sweden, and her work is largely made up of consultations with men prior to and after prostate treatments, helping them to find sexual practices that work for their bodies as they now are. This is not a straightforward task, and what solutions work vary from man to man. Much of the complexity stems, of course, from the fact that different types of treatment will produce different side effects, so depending on if a man has had radiation treatment, hormone therapy, or a surgical procedure, his body will react and recover differently.[11] But a lot of the complexity also stems from the fact that sexuality and how it is performed is very different from man to man. Even if one is asking only about a particular aspect of sexual practice—for instance, the ability to achieve a sufficiently hard erection—there are variations to consider: How is that erection going to be used? Does it need to be hard enough for anal penetration? Or just for a hand job? Or a blow job? Or to penetrate a vagina? And erections are only a part of many men's sexual repertoire. Opening up for other aspects of arousal, intimacy, orgasm, etc.,[12] in the clinical conversation can be generative, but it takes more time, and any problem will not necessarily be "solved" by the pharmaceuticals (delivered by pills, sticks, and injections) usually prescribed for impotence.

The prostate is also identified as an erotic zone in and of itself, as a node of pleasurable stimulation in many cultural narratives, even if some medical work would suggest that it is the nerves in the anal structure that lie behind that.[13] Another Swedish sexologist I interviewed said he would often mention "prostate stimulation" during consultations, either through anal penetration or by using a vibrator on the perineum. He tried to counter the common misconception that an erection happens only in the penis, and start a conversation about the entire genital region (the prostate, of course, but also the testicles, the perineum, the anus, and the pelvic muscles) as an erogenous zone. Given that patients with erectile dysfunction sometimes report being able to achieve orgasm through stimulation of the penis tip, even if the penis is not hard,[14] these other erogenous areas can be useful to remember. But for some men, it is not so much the ability to achieve orgasm itself as the actual erection that is an important way of relating to and being with other bodies: of *doing* sex with other people.

Danemalm Jägervall and another colleague of mine, Brüggemann, have done quite a bit of research into the way men experience their post-treatment bodies and post-prostatectomy sex.[15] Some of this has been with newly treated patients, some with men who have been cancer-free for ten years or more. They have interviewed men who self-identify as gay, but also heterosexual men. Much of their research has looked at how men make sense of their new bodily abilities.[16]

As part of this research, Brüggemann studied the repair work[17] strategies that men used to explain and address the side effects of their prostate cancer treatments, especially impotence. He noticed that, just as the particular side effects can vary depending on what sort of treatment one receives, so can the severity of how a man experiences those side effects vary, as can the strategies he employs to repair them. Some men attempt to return their physical body to a condition that is reminiscent of how it was before, using medical technologies or rehabilitation treatments to regain erectile capabilities. Other men are more comfortable with the idea that their bodies are ageing, and change is just something that happens to ageing bodies, explaining away the surgical effects as a part of getting older. Brüggemann noted, too, that the types of relationships a man was in, or could imagine initiating, tended to affect the way they dealt with impotence.[18] In line with other research, he has found that men who are not in a monogamous relationship—especially those who are single—may experience the negative impact of prostate cancer treatment more severely than others.[19]

Prostate cancer has been called a couple's disease, and Brüggemann's work suggests that the medical establishment could be more helpful by integrating the opportunity to engage in couples counseling for men in a relationship rather than offering only biomedical treatments for erectile dysfunction. But—he and others caution—it is necessary for healthcare practitioners to be aware of the assumptions they may be making about the man they encounter and his potential relationships. "Couple" is a complicated term. And in actuality, many men end up visiting the doctor's office on their own—maybe they don't want to ask their partner to take time off work, or don't have a relationship which assumes that the partner is a support structure for moments like this.[20] Additionally, a partner's potential response can vary. A partner may, for example, be afraid of getting prostate cancer, or maybe already have prostate issues himself. Female partners may experience being in the role of supportive partner differently.[21] Likewise, women may provide cancer care in general for their partners differently than male partners,[22] and may be more proactive in finding information about and encouraging PSA tests.[23]

Another way of dealing with the stress of a prostate cancer diagnosis, treatment, and recovery is participation in a prostate cancer survivor group. This works for some—possibly many—men, but not all. Some men may glean strength from being part of a collective focused on survivorship, or find purpose in actively helping others or lobbying for increased research into the disease.[24] But others may not. I am reminded of my colleague who had a lot to share about his PSA test experiences, but didn't want to talk about it in front of others. Not everyone feels like talking about it. Likewise, some men find the assumed heterosexual presentation many men come to these groups with uncomfortable, while others may not.[25] Prostate cancer survivor groups are vocal and visible actors on the prostate cancer scene (witness Movember; see chapter 5), but not all men want their prostate cancer to be visible, nor are they comfortable with vocalizing their ways of dealing with its side effects.

Masculinities under Threat

From the critique mentioned above about the presumed heteronormativity in prostate cancer treatment and literature, one can draw suggestions on how to be more inclusive in care provision. That is important, and I hope this book will nudge that process along. But the critique is also, for a social scientist like me, a clear indicator of the heteronormative aspects of masculinity that are shaping the cultural contours of the prostate. The prostate is still very closely associated with a heterosexual masculinity, and one which would seem to be dominated by assumed penetrative vaginal sex. As in the historical material and the diagnostic guidelines, the cultural contours of the absent prostate are being shaped and formed by how prostate cancer treatment side effects are discussed. Perhaps these shapes and forms are actually in line with many men's understandings of their prostate, their sexuality, and their health. But for many others . . . perhaps not.

Whichever masculinities we choose to associate with the prostate, however, it would seem as if masculinity in some form or another is ever-present. One psychologist I interviewed spoke about how many of his clients who had been through prostate surgery would say that they didn't feel as if they were real men anymore. (I've heard that in my interviews with men, as well, and from some partners, too. But I've also been cornered at the end of an evening and heard stories of improved sex lives and new techniques.) Rather than leaving this cliché hanging in the air during his sessions, the psychologist usually tried to get men to talk about what they meant by it. Their feelings stemmed from the loss of erection and potency, of not being able to perform. Often, this was expressed as not being able to have sex in the same way as before. The man might not feel as virile—perhaps his desire was missing, as well as the ability to have an erection. But also, the man didn't feel as strong as before. Often he felt weak and in need of help, which is not surprising given the experience of being treated for a life-threatening disease like cancer. But this weakness, this vulnerability, this need for help, is difficult to integrate into an identity based on masculine ideals of strength and self-sufficiency, not to mention the physical difficulties of erectile problems or incontinence. These impact on any human being, but they interact with masculinity in particular ways. Somewhere in our cultural imaginary, we think that strength and a strong erection are signs of being a man. If a man can no longer get an erection, what is he then? A woman? These are actual questions the psychologist hears from his clients.

Well, you might say, that's not so strange. The prostate is a male gland and prostate cancer is a man's disease. It's a common assertion,[26] and as the earlier part of this book has shown, masculinity (a very culturally contingent, specific understanding of masculinity, it should be remembered) is shaping how we understand, examine, diagnose, and treat the prostate and prostate cancer at every turn.

But what if we were to think about women's bodies with prostate cancer? Most discussions of prostate cancer, and most studies about it, tend to focus on cis male bodies, and work within a binary paradigm. But transgender women can get prostate cancer. Possibly because of the interplay between orchidectomy, hormone therapy, and hormone-related cancers, the number of transgender women with prostate cancer is probably low,[27] but they do exist. The urology profession is going to have to adapt to new routines to ensure that transgender women and nonbinary people with prostates are visible to the healthcare structures, and have access to the care they may need around urological cancers.[28] Right now, most of what little research there is into transgender women and prostate cancer tends to focus on the relationship between hormones and the development of cancer, as well as how cancer treatment options interact with other hormone treatments. There is almost nothing on how transgender women *experience* prostate cancer treatments and the side effects of these treatments, or what support structures can best help them. But one could imagine that the cultural contours of the prostate would be enrolled into those treatments and recovery processes in different ways; that focus would shift away from bodily ways of doing masculinity to ways and scripts that make trans identity intelligible, especially in healthcare settings.[29] I have not done this research yet, nor found anyone who has, but in an interview that Danemalm Jägervall conducted with a transgender woman who had survived prostate cancer, it would appear that the change in erectile and ejaculatory abilities is experienced differently by her than by many cis men. As she said in that interview, "They told me that the cancer treatment might affect my sex life, but that has never been important to me, so I took it in my stride."[30]

This is *one* interview. It is not a sufficient basis for any generalizations. But it does let us peek under the lid a little bit and see how, sometimes, our physical abilities are entangled with sexuality, and sexuality is entangled with our self-identity, and our self-identity is entangled with social expectations, "appropriate" scripts, norms, institutional structures, and the material world . . . and that these entanglements are *messy*. They are not straightforward, and they are not the same for everyone. When cis male prostate cancer survivors, straight, gay, or bi, wonder if they are still real[31] men because of the loss of ejaculation and erectile changes, their concerns are stemming from that messy entanglement which produces expectations of those abilities in connection with culturally contingent masculinities.

But what fascinates *me* most of all is that this messy muddle of damaged or repaired masculine identities is blamed on the prostate—a prostate that often isn't even there. Absent, but oh, so present.

Anxiety, Angst, Torment, and . . . a Lot of Talking

I mentioned above that this research was inspired by medical texts that would say things like: "It is probably his prostate that is haunting him," or "The prostate—a constant torment," without really being clear what the prostate was actually doing, or why it had gradually become a torment. The prostate could be blamed for a lot of diffuse, hard to define or diagnose problems, especially with the term "prostatitis." Sometimes it seemed as if it was taking the blame for medical problems associated with masculinity, ageing, sex, and urination that we are not really sure how to diagnose or treat. But sometimes it was very clear that the prostate was diseased and needed to be treated, even removed. In these cases—cancer being the most obvious—the prostate is indeed a source of constant torment, haunting the man long after it is gone.

But whether it is gone or still in the body, what the prostate "is" can be very complicated because in different discourses it "is" a messy entanglement of glands, muscles, hormones, disease, and health, but also sexuality, sexual practices, understandings of masculinity, sporting activities, cultural events, social expectations. . . . It is made known in our built environment in different ways—where toilets are available, for example, or which facilities have receptacles for the disposal of used incontinence pads—and through the interactions with healthcare infrastructures and binary paradigms that form the basis of specialist fields. On top of that, our modern understandings are at least slightly tinged by the historical development of knowledge about the prostate. As a neuroscientist friend of mine has observed in her work on surgical procedures and the brain, "The world writes on the whole body."[32] To understand how that body is doing, we also have to understand how the world is writing on it.

I hope this book has opened up some thoughts about what the prostate is, not only what doctors think might be wrong with it. I hope it has provided a few insights into how, and maybe even why, the prostate features so prominently in the *zeitgeist*. And above all, I hope this book has convinced you that knowledge about the prostate is not confined to biomedical knowledge, even if it is to medicine that we first turn when confronted with possible prostate issues. The prostate—and the pathologies associated with it as it ages, in particular prostate cancer—has seeped far beyond anatomy books, blood-testing laboratories, and surgical theaters. Today, the (diseased) prostate is prominently positioned in our cultural imaginary and terrifies many men, young and old alike. And their partners, children, friends. In some discourses, the (undiseased) prostate is also prominent, working as a node of sexual pleasure. What the prostate does, where it is located, and what might actually go biomedically wrong with it is often, rightfully, very important to many people. But the prostate also appears frequently in conversations tangential to sexuality, masculinity, and ageing. What the prostate does in our body is bound up with what it does for our understandings of ourselves, as we age.

Bodies with prostates are not all the same. The transgender woman's response to prostate cancer treatment showed this poignantly, but even without that example, it should be clear by now that "man" is not a natural, stable, homogeneous category, even for cis men.[33] To complicate things more, men are relational beings, becoming who they are in their interactions with others, be those colleagues, family, friends, lovers. Their identities are intimately entangled with those relations. Inevitably, the prostate also becomes enrolled in this entanglement of relations. Its health is intimately associated with the health of the man, his social connections, and the worlds he inhabits. Had I written that about an aspect of a woman's reproductive system, it would hardly seem controversial, given the last fifty years of women's health research and activism into which the statement would be embedded. Perhaps it is time to turn the wisdom of these conversations to men's bodies, as well.

The prostate is not only a source of constant physical torment. It is a cause of much anxiety. But what anxiety, specifically? Is it the worry of not being able to get it up (for whatever purposes one wants it to be up to)? Is it the connection between erections and manhood? Changing sexual abilities? Or changing masculinities? Or is it the worry of being constantly tormented by needing to "pee like an old man," as one of my informants called it? Or ageing in general? Or of dying from cancer?

All of these anxieties—about sexuality, masculinity, ageing, health, and death—are shaping how we think about the prostate. And how we talk about it, diagnose it, treat it, and treat bodies who have lost it. When I think about these anxieties, I am slightly more forgiving of the response I got when I called an old college friend to tell him I had received a long-term grant to do research into the prostate. He managed a forced "congratulations" between gritted teeth, then said he didn't really want to talk about the prostate. Little did I know then that in the intervening years, *he* may not have wanted to talk about it, but a lot of other people (fortunately) did. From social conversations and research interviews with men who were worried about it, treating it, or missing it, to interviews with medical professionals whose careers have helped those men, I have found myself awash in conversations about that small, walnut-shaped gland. For a topic of conversation one often tries to avoid, the prostate is surprisingly present—even in its absence—in our cultural imaginary.

Afterthoughts

Academic research in the medical humanities can contribute to our understanding of our bodies, our subjectivities (who we are as people), and our health and illness, in several different ways. By studying the interactions between medical knowledge (and knowledge- making practices) and the bodies and subjectivities they engage, this work can show how medicine's practices affect the experience of being ill, but also the experience of being healthy. Medicine impacts on our diseased existence, and on what it means to be well. By applying humanities and social science approaches (methods, theories, and—importantly—understandings of what constitutes legitimate, useful data) we are also able to expand questions about health and illness to include data beyond the biomedical paradigm. I am not saying that biomedical data is irrelevant, but I am suggesting that it gives only a partial view of health or illness. By extending a research approach to include other data (historical material, visual representations, the material world and how things in it produce particular understanding,

and also literary and cultural narratives, patient experiences, expectations, dreams, and whispers about the
hope of health), and by using analytical methods drawn
from the social sciences and the humanities that analyze these data and contextualize them in historical,
cultural, and organizational contexts, we can frame and
then execute studies which engage the person and the
world, rather than only the biomedical processes of an
organism.

I hope that this book does that for the prostate, and
for the well-being of those people whose bodies have
or have had a prostate. I have drawn on many sources
of data which are generally not used in biomedical
research about the prostate. These include in-depth,
open-ended interviews with patients and practitioners,
material from historical archives, notes on social trends
and media representations of prostate issues, and analysis of the discursive framings and turns in medical texts.
In my work, and in the research projects from which it
draws, my team and I have used these sources to show
how knowledge-making processes about the prostate are
intimately related to social understandings of masculinity, sexuality, and ageing, both historically and today. I
have also been attentive to how the physical, material
elements of medical approaches to the prostate—how
it is examined, what techniques and tests are used, and
within which medical disciplines—affect the patients
and the prostate diagnosis they can receive. By engaging theoretical discussions and tools about men's health

and masculinity, but also about medicalization, the sexed and gendered body, the way the body is experienced, patient subjectivities (especially social and vulnerable ones), multiple ontologies, epistemological critiques, and the absent–present body,[1] I have tried to show how the prostate is present, sometimes even when it is absent, in many conversations about what it means to be a man. I read the material in this book as also showing that this discursive presence is pervasive, but not immutable. Its contours can generate particular ghosts which can haunt, but those contours are not necessarily the same in all contexts (they are contingent), and can therefore be contested and changed.

These finding are in line with work in the medical humanities, and though I wouldn't claim to be developing any of its particular theoretical arguments further, I am indebted to previous work in the field in order to make these points. I've used many of the interdisciplinary tools that the medical humanities espouse. Perhaps this book's contribution is to present an example of how an interdisciplinary medical humanities study can engage a diverse team of researchers and a wide range of conversations to address a particular topic from many angles.

But why bother? What is the real-world impact of research like this? Well, I hope this book can give some concrete suggestions as to how practitioners and patients can think about the prostate as it is engaged in different conversations about health and well-being today. I have looked at how the prostate is medicalized, why and when it becomes a problem, and how the problematic prostate is experienced by, above all, the men whose body it resides in or is taken out of, but also those who are tasked with knowing and treating it.

One thing that has become clear is that not all prostates are diseased, especially over the life course. Nor are all prostates a source of torment. Some may even be a source of pleasure. And regardless of how they are experienced, they serve a purpose for healthy reproduction. Yet the prostate has assumed—or been given—the role of a lurking antagonist about to threaten lives at every turn. It then follows that the prostate (as a discursive node and a pathologized gland) becomes a constant torment that can haunt a man. This can explain the figure of speech that had confounded me at the beginning of my project. The prostate becomes a way to speak about the ageing male body by simultaneously pathologizing it, by engaging a constant fear of ageing, cancer, and death. Yes, the prostate is sometimes truly ill, and needs to be treated. But there is a lot more happening within those discussion, as well.

Social science work on the medicalized female body has shown how the uterus, pregnancy, and menopause have been medicalized and simultaneously therewith used to pathologize female bodies, turning them (and in particular sex, reproduction, and ageing) into sites for medical control and profit.[2] A lot of the analytical work done in this project was informed by feminist theory; in

particular, studies of women's health issues and the relationship between academic study and health activism.[3]
Observations from this body of literature can also throw
useful light on what is happening to the prostate. Lessons could be drawn from it on how this knowledge has
been transformed into campaigns that demand medical care aimed at women's health and well-being. These
campaigns, and the changes to healthcare provision
they have instigated during the last forty years, are ben-
efiting women around the world. Activists for prostate
care could learn from them. Movember and other campaigns and prostate cancer survivor groups have already
learned much from breast cancer survivor mobilization.
But there are other lessons that can be shared across the
divide between women's and men's health. One of these
may be found in what is sometimes called the "epistemological critique": the demand that medicine take
into consideration the way the person knows their own
body (a patient's lived experience) and engage patient/
person- generated knowledge about health, and about
what it means to be healthy to that individual.[4] In this
research, one can find acknowledgement that medical
knowledge about our bodies and pathologies is colored
by understandings and expectations of socially appropriate behavior, especially when sex and reproduction
are involved, as well as gendered understandings of
appropriate behavior—historically and today. Pointing out the parallels this research reveals between discussions of women's bodies and discussions about this

prostate reminds us that knowledge can be contested from both within and outside of medicine. It means acknowledging how seriously medical treatments of our body can affect our physical and emotional well-being (positively and negatively), including our relationships with others and our ways of being in the world. And it means demanding that patients are involved in making truly informed decisions about their health.

I recognize that doing so is hard. And complex. And not something everybody wants to do (or should be expected to do, for that matter). It requires listening and talking, from both the patient and the doctor. And it means imagining and discussing health beyond the biomedical data recorded in a patient file—perhaps even with professionals other than medical doctors. The examples and cases in this book would suggest that we need to get better at those conversations, in the clinic and outside it, at the personal and at the policy level, when it comes to prostate health. I hope the research I and my team have produced can further—or at least encourage—those conversations.

Acknowledgments

This book is based on a long-term, multi-sited research project that engaged researchers from different academic fields, departments, and universities. I am so grateful to the "Constant Torment" team: for all of their thorough and dedicated work, of course, but also for all of the joy and curiosity we shared through the course of this project. Thank you Elin Björk, Maria Björkman, Jelmer Brüggemann, Carina Danemalm Jägervall, Jenny Gleisner, Sonja Jerak-Zuiderent, Oscar Maldonado Castañeda, and Alma Persson! Many of the results reported on here are theirs. The mistakes and misinterpretations are mine.

The seminar group "Body, Knowledge, Subjectivity" at the Department of Thematic Studies provided the social and theoretical home for the work we did in the project—and challenged us to see our material in new and different ways. Thank you for giving feedback so generously and warmly, especially Nimmo Elmi, Hannah Grankvist, Alex Gribble, Lisa Guntram, Ruben Hordijk, Alexandra Kapeller, Corinna Kruse, Sofia

Morberg Jämterud, Toby Odland, and Kristin Zeiler. I also received valuable input from members of the Center for Medical Humanities and Bioethics at Linköping University, as well as from other colleagues who came with important insights at critical times, including Catelijne Coopmans, Björn Berglin, Boel Berner, Bettina Bock von Wülfingen, Anna Bredström, Mark Elam, Kathrin Friedrich, Matias Garzón, Henrik Kjölhede, Lisa Lindén, Piotr Maroń, Ralph Peeker, Anna Storm, Kristina Trygg, James Tycast, Else Vogel, Richard Wassersug, Steve Woolgar, and Teun Zuiderent-Jerak. And thank you to Mo Aufderhaar, Ka Schmitz, and Oliver Eberhard at Pudelskern.

Much of my own work has involved in-depth interviews with men who in some way or another are deeply engaged with the prostate: as potential patients, former patients, or professionals whose work attempts to help those with prostate problems. Thank you for being so open with your experiences and reflections! And, of course, thank you to those of you in my daily life who have put up with my decidedly odd and oddly decided fascination with this gland for so many years.

Thanks are also due to Nina Rehnqvist and the Young Academy of Sweden, especially Gustaf Edgren, Anna Kjällström, Annika Moberg, Helena Rosik, and Anna Wetterbom, as well as the invited speakers Olof Akre, Kjell Asplund, and Kristin Zeiler, and guests for providing the opportunity to facilitate the scientific salon described in chapter 5. This was the highlight of my research project!

Our work has also benefited from generous access to historical archive material about the prostate from the Hagströmer Medico-Historical Library, the Medical History Museum and Library, University of Zurich (now the Archive of the History of Medicine and Institute of Evolutionary Medicine, University of Zurich), and the Semmelweis University Library. I've also been generously assisted by Carina Danemalm Jägervall, Patricia Glowinski, Ylva Huge, and Reidar Källström for help with images.

Funding for this research came from the Swedish Research Council, projects "Det ständiga gisslet. Diskursiva konturer av den åldrande prostatan" (Dnr 2013-8048) and "Genus och medicinska simulatorer" (Dnr 2012-5198), and from Riksbankens Jubileumsfond, for archival work in Budapest. I am also thankful for institutional support from Linköping University.

And, of course, thank you to Pam Bertram and Gillian Beaumont for help with final edits, and to my acquisitions editor, Matt Browne, for believing so steadfastly and waiting so patiently.

Notes

Introduction

1. R. Solnit, *Storming the Gates of Paradise: Landscapes for Politics* (Oakland: University of California Press, 2007).

2. I am not a medical doctor. This book does not contain medical advice.

3. For recent examples, see: https://www.sporthoj.com/forum/show thread.php?269579-Svårt-att-kissa; https://prostatype.se/prostata-test -pa-dig-sjalv/

4. As it was described, for example, in A-C. Kinn et al., *Prostata— mannens ständiga gissel* (Södertälje: Astra Sverige, 1997).

5. Here I am thinking of S. Sontag, *Illness as Metaphor* (New York: Farrar, Straus & Giroux, 1978), of course. But I am also thinking with scholars in feminist technoscience studies. Much of the work on the role of tropes in the production of scientific knowledge has been inspired by D. Haraway, *Modest_Witness@Second_Millennium. FemaleMan©_Meets_OncoMouse™: Feminism and Technoscience* (New York: Routledge, 1997). Martin's analysis of metaphors in fertilization research is also a staple of this approach; see E. Martin, "The Egg and the Sperm: How Science Has Constructed a Romance Based on Stereotypical Male–Female Roles," *Signs* 16, no. 3 (1991): 485–501. N. Oudshoorn, *Beyond the Natural Body* (London: Routledge, 1994) has also been inspiring. However, throughout I will also be working

with ideas presented by A. Mol, *The Body Multiple* (Durham: Duke University Press, 2002) and C. Thompson, *Making Parents: The Ontological Choreography of Reproductive Technologies* (Cambridge, MA: MIT Press, 2005), who integrate the material aspects of the body and the technologies of knowing it with an analysis of the metaphors and discourses used to describe it.

6. I use the term historical here to reflect the fact that I will be engaging in some historical work and archival material about a specific object, the prostate, but I call my work a cultural biography rather than a social history, inspired by Appadurai's distinction between the study of specific things (biographies) and larger, historical ebbs and flows in the shifting meanings of a class or type (social histories); see A. Appadurai, ed., *The Social Life of Things: Commodities in Cultural Perspective* (New York: Cambridge University Press, 1986), 34.

7. This is a field that, among other things, takes seriously the idea that the material world, our understandings about it, and our ways and practices of making knowledge are extremely relevant to what knowledge is made, where, and by whom. I tend to draw heavily on work that discusses the relational agency of humans and non-humans involved in producing knowledge about the world: for example, Haraway, *Modest_Witness*; K. Barad, *Meeting the Universe Halfway* (Durham: Duke University Press, 2007); L. Suchman, *Human Machine Reconfigurations: Plans and Situation Actions*, 2nd ed. (Cambridge: Cambridge University Press, 2007); A. M. Mol, *The Body Multiple: Ontology in Medical Practice* (Durham: Duke University Press, 2002).

8. I. Kopytoff, "The Cultural Biography of Things: Commoditization as Process," in Appadurai, ed., *The Social Life of Things*, 64–91; C. Gosden and Y. Marshall, "The Cultural Biography of Objects," *World Archaeology* 31, no. 2 (1999): 169–178.

9. Cf. J. Hoskins, *Biographical Objects: How Things Tell the Story of People's Lives* (London: Routledge, 1998).

10. L. Daston, ed., *Biographies of Scientific Objects* (Chicago: University of Chicago Press, 2000), 13.

11. Daston, *Biographies of Scientific Objects*, 9.

12. Barad, *Meeting the Universe Halfway*.

13. Solnit, *Storming the Gates of Paradise*.

14. B. Latour, "On the Partial Existence of Existing and Non-Existing Objects," in Daston, *Biographies of Scientific Objects*, 250.

15. Here I am taking a cue from the epistemological critique found in research on women's health and its historically porous border to activism; see K. Davis, *The Making of* Our Bodies, Ourselves*: How Feminism Travels across Borders* (Durham: Duke University Press, 2007); B. Ehrenreich and D. English, *Witches, Midwives and Nurses: A History of Women Healers* (New York: Feminist Press at the City University of New York, 1973); S. Epstein, *Inclusion: The Politics of Difference in Medical Research* (Chicago: University of Chicago Press, 2007); M. Murphy, *Seizing the Means of Reproduction: Entanglements of Feminism, Health and Technoscience* (Durham: Duke University Press, 2012); N. Tuana, "The Speculum of Ignorance: The Women's Health Movement and Epistemologies of Ignorance," *Hypatia* 21, no. 3 (2006): 1–19. This type of academic work we can do in the medical humanities; it is a contribution the medical humanities research can make to our empirical fields.

16. A person who was assigned male at birth and whose gender identity is male.

17. I reach back to I. Illich, *Limits to Medicine/Medical Nemesis: The Expropriation of Health* (London: Marion Boyars, 1975), here, but also even further. In some of the early medical sociology, e.g., M. Balint, *The Doctor, His Patient and the Illness* (London: Pitman, 1957); H. S. Becker et al., *Boys in White: Student Culture in Medical School* (New Brunswick, NJ: Transaction Publishers, 1961); R. L. Coser, "Alienation and the Social Structure: Case Analysis of a Hospital," in *The Hospital in Modern Society: Eleven Stories of the Hospital Today*, ed. E. Freidson (London: Free Press of Glencoe, 1963); J. Eaton and R. Weil, *Culture and Mental Disorders* (Glencoe, IL: Free Press, 1955); R. Fox, *Experiment Perilous: Physician and Patients Facing the Unknown* (Glencoe, IL: Free Press, 1959); Freidson, *The Hospital in Modern Society*; T. Parsons, *Social*

Structure and Dynamic Process: The Case of the Modern Medical Practice (London: Routledge, 1951), I find inspiration in the wide-eyed attempt to understand the relationships between patients, doctors, society, medical therapies, and the production of knowledge (also L. Fleck "The Problem of Epistemology" (1936), in *Cognition and Fact: Materials on Ludwig Fleck*, ed. R. S. Cohen (Dordrecht: Reidel, 1986). In this scholarship I see medicine beginning to be an object of study rather than a fount of knowledge.

18. Medical knowledge—like all knowledge—changes as it moves through time and place, belying the foundational premise of evidence-based medicine; see S. Timmermans and B. Marc, *The Gold Standard: The Challenge of Evidence-Based Medicine and Standardization in Healthcare* (Philadelphia: Temple University Press, 2003); E. Johnson et al., *Glocal Pharma: International Brands and the Imagination of Local Masculinity* (London: Routledge, 2016).

19. This is sometimes called the second wave of the medical humanities, and is a rapidly growing area of research; see A. Whitehead and A. Woods, eds., *The Edinburgh Companion to the Critical Medical Humanities* (Edinburgh: Edinburgh University Press, 2016); W. Viney et al., "Critical Medical Humanities: Embracing Entanglement, Taking Risks," *Medical Humanities* 41 (2015): 2–7.

20. M. Björkman, ed., *Prostatan—det ständiga gisslet? Mannen och prostatan I kultur, medicin och historia* (Lund: Nordic Academic Press, 2018).

21. Haraway, *Modest_Witness*.

22. In accordance with Swedish research ethics policy, a joint application was made for those parts of the project (interviews with current or past patients) which were deemed relevant for ethics board appraisal. The same ethical approach to interviews with practitioners was applied, even though this did not require formal approval in the Swedish system. Approval was granted in the decision *Regionala etikprövningsnämnden i Linköping, avdelning för prövning av övrig forskning,* dnr 2016/167–31.

23. This also became an issue when I made an informational film with some of my informants, reproducing their biomedical understandings of the prostate; see Chapter 1. In these discussions we were inspired by conversations with Teun Zuiderent-Jerak, who has written on the intricacies of doing research and making interventions on and with a field; see T. Zuiderent-Jerak, *Situated Intervention: Sociological Experiments in Health Care* (Cambridge, MA: MIT Press, 2015).

Chapter 1

1. https://www.youtube.com/watch?v=pZwvrxVavnQ

2. https://www.youtube.com/watch?v=3DPVAGCylMA

3. G. Einstein et al., "The Gendered Ovary: Whole Body Effects of Oophorectomy," *Canadian Journal of Nursing Research* 44, no. 3 (2012): 7–17.

4. One of these is phenomenology, especially as used in medical humanities research; for example, D. Leder, *The Absent Body* (Chicago: University of Chicago Press, 1990), and in the discussion of the pre-reflexive body in K. Zeiler, "A Phenomenological Analysis of Bodily Self-Awareness in the Experience of Pain and Pleasure: On Dys-Appearance and Eu-Appearance," *Medical Health Care and Philosophy* 13, no. 4 (2010): 333–342.

5. *die weibliche Prostata.* Some people say that the G-spot is the female equivalent of the prostate, and sometimes this area is called Skene's gland. There have even been a few cases of "female prostate cancer" in bodies with a uterus (Thum et al., "[Female Prostate Cancer?]," *Pathologe* 38, no 5 [2017]: 448–450), but in most medical books, men have prostates, not women.

6. There are many good resources on the net that can give more information like this. For example, U.S. National Library of Medicine has good on-line information about the anatomy of the prostate; for further details, their website is at: www.ncbi.nlm.nih.gov

7. This has been well documented by medical historians like L. Jordanova, *Nature Displayed: Gender, Science and Medicine 1760–1820*

(London: Longman, 1999), 189 (especially her discussion of the cultural, material, and technical relationships between art, anatomy, the mythical, and the symbolic, pp. 193–194); and S. Jülich, "The Making of a Best-Selling Book on Reproduction: Lennart Nilsson's *A Child Is Born*," *Bulletin of the History of Medicine* 89, no. 3 (2015): 491–525. There are also interesting cultural critiques of visualization practices and computer technologies; for example, J. van Dijck, *The Transparent Body: A Cultural Analysis of Medical Imaging* (Seattle: University of Washington Press, 2015); K. Friedrich, "From 'Imaging 2.0' to 'Imaging 3.0'," in *Scientific Knowledge and the Transgression of Boundaries*, ed. B-J. Krings, H. Rodríguez, and A. Schleisiek (Berlin: Verlag für Sozialwissenschaften, 2016). Here one also finds work on visualization technologies' relationship to gender; see C. Waldby, *The Visible Human Project: Informatic Bodies and Posthuman Medicine* (London: Routledge, 2000). Similar concerns about the practices of representation can be found among practitioners within the field of visualization; see M. Meyer and J. Dykes, "Criteria for Rigor in Visualization Design Study," *IEEE Transactions on Visualization and Computer Graphics* 26, no. 1 (2020): 87–97.

8.   Statens Beredning för Medicinsk och Social Utvärdering (SBU), *Godartad prostataförstoring med avflödeshinder. En systematisk litteraturöversikt*, Swedish Council on Health Technology Assessment, 2011, 220.

9.   Lehrtafel Anatomisches Institut der Universität Zürich, Zeichner: E. Brändli 30.09.1943. Archiv für Medizingeschichte Universität Zürich, Signatur IN 25 Nr. 417.

10.   This was closed in 2015; the collection is now part of the Institute of Evolutionary Medicine.

11.   Archiv für Medizingeschichte Universität Zürich, Inv. No. 1083.

Chapter 2

1.   R. Shotwell, "Animals, Pictures, and Skeletons: Andreas Vesalius's Reinvention of the Public Anatomy Lesson," *Journal of the History of Medicine and Allied Sciences* 71, no. 1 (2015): 1–18.

2. D. Shackley, "A Century of Prostatic Surgery," *BJU International* 83, no. 7 (1999): 776.

3. Shackley, "A Century of Prostatic Surgery," 776.

4. F. J. Marx and A. Karenberg, "Uro-Words Making History: Ureter and Urethra," *The Prostate* 70 (2010): 952–958.

5. Marx and Karenberg, "Uro-Words Making History," 209.

6. For more on the history of anatomy theaters and dissection practices, see Shotwell, "Animals, Pictures, and Skeletons" 1–18; C. Klestinec, "A History of Anatomy Theaters in Sixteenth-Century Padua," *Journal of the History of Medicine and Allied Sciences* 59, no. 3 (2004) 375–412. For cultural aspects of the knowledge gained from dissection practices, see L. Schiebinger, *Nature's Body: Gender in the Making of Modern Science* (Boston: Beacon Press, 1993); for more recent controversies about dissection, see S. Burrell and G. Gill, "The Liverpool Cholera Epidemic of 1832 and Anatomical Dissection—Medical Mistrust and Civil Unrest," *Journal of the History of Medicine and Allied Sciences* 60, no. 4 (2005): 475–498.

7. Marx and Karenberg, "Uro-Words Making History," 209.

8. Marx and Karenberg, "Uro-Words Making History," 210; J. Goddard, "The Prostate in Five Pictures," *Journal of Clinical Urology* 12, no. 15 (2019): 4–8.

9. Marx and Karenberg, "Uro-Words Making History," 210; see also H. K. Valier, *A History of Prostate Cancer, Men and Medicine* (London: Palgrave Macmillan, 2016), esp. chapter 2, "The Problematic Prehistory of Prostate Cancer."

10. Marx and Karenberg, "Uro-Words Making History," 211.

11. G. Phillips, in *Prostatic Hypertrophy from Every Surgical Standpoint by George M. Phillips M.D. and Forty Distinguished Authorities*, ed. S. C. Martin, Jr. (St. Louis: AJOD Company, Medical Publishers, 1903), 19.

12. Phillips, *Prostatic Hypertrophy*, 20.

13. S. D. O'Shea, "'A Plea for the Prostate': Doctors, Prostate Dysfunction, and Male Sexuality in Late 19th- and Early 20th-Century Canada," *Canadian Bulletin of Medical History* 29, no. 1 (2012): 7–27.

14. Phillips, *Prostatic Hypertrophy*, 24.

15. O'Shea, "'A Plea for the Prostate'"; see also A. McLaren, *Impotence: A Cultural History* (Chicago: University of Chicago Press, 2007).

16. O'Shea, "'A Plea for the Prostate'."

17. S. Ciechanowski, *Prostatic Hypertrophy: Anatomical Researches on the So-Called "Prostatic Hypertrophy" and Allied Processes in the Bladder and Kidneys* (New York: Pelton, 1938), 138; J. Vander Veer, *Clinical Aspects of the Enlarged Prostate, With a Review of 67 Cases*, reprinted from the *New York State Journal of Medicine* (1909), 3; H. Young, *Studies on Hypertrophy and Cancer of the Prostate*, Johns Hopkins Hospital Reports Vol. XIV (Baltimore: Johns Hopkins University Press, 1906), 44.

18. Vander Veer, *Clinical Aspects of the Enlarged Prostate*, 3–4; Young, *Studies on Hypertrophy and Cancer of the Prostate*, 46.

19. Young, *Studies on Hypertrophy and Cancer of the Prostate*, 46.

20. Vander Veer, *Clinical Aspects of the Enlarged Prostate*, 3.

21. Phillips, *Prostatic Hypertrophy*, 52, 55, 110, 127.

22. Phillips, *Prostatic Hypertrophy*, 24.

23. Phillips, *Prostatic Hypertrophy*, 24, 52, 12.

24. Phillips, *Prostatic Hypertrophy*, 24, 52, 128.

25. O'Shea, "'A Plea for the Prostate'"; Phillips, *Prostatic Hypertrophy*, 24.

26. This is not a historical anomaly. There was a similar product, designed to treat incontinence, reviewed in the Swedish medical journal in 1999 (M. Fall, "Urininkontinens hos mannen—ett försummat problem?," *Läkartidningen* 96, no. 18 [1999]: 2227–2231), and one of the men I interviewed in 2017 had been treated with electricity to shrink his prostate.

27. H. L. Kretschmer, "Electrosection of the Prostate," Chicago: Presbyterian Hospital, 1932(?), 3.

28. Shackley, "A Century of Prostatic Surgery"; O'Shea, "'A Plea for the Prostate'."

29. L. Fleck, "The Problem of Epistemology" (1936), in *Cognition and Fact: Materials on Ludwik Fleck*, ed. R. S. Cohen and T. Schnelle (Dordrecht: Reidel, 1986), 89; K. Wailoo, *Drawing Blood: Technology and Disease Identity in Twentieth-Century America* (Baltimore: Johns Hopkins University Press, 1997).

30. E. Björk, "Att bota en prostata. Kastrering som behandlingsmetod för prostatahypertrofi 1893–1910," PhD diss., Linköping University 2019, 29.

31. Björk, "Att bota en prostata," 1.

32. Shackley, "A Century of Prostatic Surgery," 778.

33. Björk, "Att bota en prostata," 1.

34. This is a huge field. One could start with, for example, S. Gilbert and S. Gubar, *The Madwoman in the Attic: The Woman Writer and the Nineteenth-Century Literary Imagination* (New Haven: Yale University Press, 1979); S. Arnaud, *On Hysteria: The Invention of a Medical Category between 1670 and 1820* (Chicago: University of Chicago Press, 2015); G. Walton, "Hysteria, as Affected by Removal of the Ovaries," *Boston Medical and Surgical Journal* 110, no. 23 (1884): 529; S. Rodriguez, *Female Circumcision and Clitoridectomy in the United States: A History of a Medical Treatment* (Rochester, NY: Boydell & Brewer, 2018); S. Frampton, *Belly-Rippers, Surgical Innovation and the Ovariotomy Controversy* (London: Palgrave Macmillan, 2018); O. Moscucci, *The Science of Woman: Gynaecology and Gender in England, 1800–1929* (Cambridge: Cambridge University Press, 1993); K. Johannison, *Den mörka kontinenten* (Stockholm: Norstedts, 1994).

35. Björk, "Att bota en prostata," 31.

36. Björk, "Att bota en prostata," 269.

37. H. Thompson, *The Diseases of the Prostate: Their Pathology and Treatment* (London: J & A. Churchill, 1873), 117; quoted in M. Björkman and A. Persson, "What's in a Gland? Sexuality, Reproduction, and the Prostate in Early Twentieth-Century Medicine," *Gender and History* 32, no. 3 (2020): 621–636; and E. Björk, "Att bota en prostata," 280.

38. Phillips, *Prostatic Hypertrophy*, 106; quoted in Björkman and Persson, "What's in a Gland?," 626.

39. For a detailed study of the development of knowledge about hormones and their use in medical treatments, see N. Oudshoorn, *Beyond the Natural Body* (London: Routledge, 1994). For a discussion on connections between this knowledge, surgical practices, and masculinity, see C. Sengoopta, *The Most Secret Quintessence of Life: Sex, Glands, and Hormones, 1850–1950* (Chicago: University of Chicago Press, 2006).

40. Björk, "Att bota en prostata," 272.

41. Björk, "Att bota en prostata," 281.

42. This was contested; see Ciechanowski, *Prostatic Hypertrophy*, 115.

43. For an overview of this, see O'Shea, "'A Plea for the Prostate'."

44. Björkman and Persson, "What's in a Gland?," 627.

45. Unsigned, "Hypertrophy of the Prostate and Gay Attire," *Urologic and Cutaneous Review* 28 (1924): 251–253.

46. G. W. Overall, *A Synopsis*, 25, quoted in Björkman and Persson, "What's in a Gland?," 630.

47. J. Polkey, "Incomplete Late Results after Supra-Pubic Prostatectomy," *Urologic and Cutaneous Review* 30 (1926): 65–74; quoted in Björkman and Persson, "What's in a Gland?," 626.

48. A tendency that has been noted in current medical practices, too; see D. Rosenfeld and C. Faircloth's groundbreaking book *Medicalized Masculinities* (Philadelphia: Temple University Press, 2006).

49. Björkman and Persson, "What's in a Gland?," 629.

50. Sengoopta, *The Most Secret Quintessence of Life*; McLaren, *Impotence*.

51. Vander Veer, *Clinical Aspects of the Enlarged Prostate*, 3.

52. Kretschmer, "Prostatic Obstruction," 17.

53. Kretschmer, "Prostatic Obstruction," 5. As Porter, who has studied the creation and maintenance of stable mortality rates by American life insurance companies, notes: "Scientific objects are not made only by scientists. Especially when we look to research involving potential use in a military, industrial, commercial, medical, agricultural, educational, regulatory, political, or bureaucratic setting, we see that they are shaped by the interests and expectations of diverse actors" (T. Porter, "Life Insurance, Medical Testing, and the Management of Mortality," in *Biographies of Scientific Objects*, ed. L. Daston [Chicago: University of Chicago Press 2000], 226).

54. Björk, "Att bota en prostata," 270.

55. Björk, "Att bota en prostata," 282.

56. Björk, "Att bota en prostata," 272.

57. Björk, "Att bota en prostata," 282.

58. C. F. Heyns and D. P. de Klerk, "Pharmaceutical Management of Benign Prostatic Hyperplasia," in *Notes from Prostatic Disorders*, ed. D. Paulson (London: Lea & Febiger, 1989), 204.

59. Heyns and de Klerk, "Pharmaceutical Management," 204–231.

60. And given that medicine is also social, what work is being done when I separate it out as its own element in that question? I am invoking an understanding of it as separate from the social to indicate the underlying materiality of the body, but this separation does more than that—it produces it as separate, and that is perhaps more emphatic than I would like.

61. Vander Veer, *Clinical Aspects of the Enlarged Prostate*, 3.

62. Phillips, *Prostatic Hypertrophy*, 75, 144.

63. Phillips, *Prostatic Hypertrophy*, cited in Björkman and Persson, "What's in a Gland?," 627.

64. Phillips, *Prostatic Hypertrophy*, 19.

65. C. Benninghaus, "Beyond Constructivism: Gender, Medicine, and the Early History of Sperm Analysis, Germany 1970–1900," *Gender and History* 24 (2012): 647–676; McLaren, *Impotence*, 106.

66. Björk, "Att bota en prostata," 213–238.

67. Björk, "Att bota en prostata," 213–238; Phillips, *Prostatic Hypertrophy*, 75.

68. Ciechanowski, *Prostatic Hypertrophy*, 138; Vander Veer, *Clinical Aspects of the Enlarged Prostate*, 3; Young, *Studies on Hypertrophy and Cancer of the Prostate*, 44.

69. E. Johnson, *Refracting through Technologies: Bodies, Medical Technologies and Norms* (London: Routledge, 2019).

70. For the praxiography which details how this happens, see A. M. Mol, *The Body Multiple: Ontology in Medical Practice* (Durham: Duke University Press, 2002).

71. D. Leder, *The Absent Body* (Chicago: University of Chicago Press, 1990).

Chapter 3

1. https://adage.com/videos/flomax-biking/592

2. https://www.youtube.com/watch?v=EU0WR-IJKmg

3. Expensive racing bikes, white-water kayaking, and golf all have overtones of class and race, especially in the US and UK contexts from which these advertisements came. Similar imaginaries have been found in Viagra advertisements in Sweden; see C. Åsberg and E. Johnson, "Viagra Selfhood: Pharmaceutical Advertising and the Visual Formations of Swedish Masculinity," in *Glocal Pharma: International Brands and the Imagination of Local Masculinities*, ed. E. Johnson with E. Sjögren and C. Åsberg (London: Routledge, 2016), 88–98.

4. For others, see Johnson et al., *Glocal Pharma*.

5. American Urological Association (AUA), "American Urological Association Guideline: Management of Benign Prostatic Hyperplasia (BPH), (Revised)" (Linthicum, MD: American Urological Association, 2010); J. Foster et al., "Surgical Management of Lower Urinary Tract Symptoms Attributed to Benign Prostatic Hyperplasia. AUA Guideline" (Linthicum, MD: American Urological Association, 2019).

6. This argument is in line with Mol's discussion of how bodies and their pathologies are enacted in particular ways (called practices) while working with technologies, which makes the idea of a cultural biography slightly more complex. It is not just a multitude of voices and sources that I would want to access; it means that the object(s) they are describing become multiple, as well. As Mol says, "It is possible to refrain from understanding objects as the central points of focus of different people's perspectives. It is possible to understand them instead as things manipulated in practices. If we do this—if instead of bracketing the practices in which objects are handled we foreground them—this has far-reaching effects. Reality multiplies." A. M. Mol, *The Body Multiple: Ontology in Medical Practice* (Durham: Duke University Press, 2002), 5.

7. J. Kellogg Parsons, "Modifiable Risk Factors for Benign Prostatic Hyperplasia and Lower Urinary Tract Symptoms: New Approaches to Old Problems," *Journal of Urology* 178, no. 2 (2007): 395.

8. A bit of a philosophical conundrum. See G. Canguilhem, *On the Normal and the Pathological* (London: Kluwer Academic Publishers, 1978).

9. Statens Beredning för Medicinsk och Social Utvärdering (SBU), *Godartad prostataförstoring med avflödeshinder. En systematisk litteraturöversikt* (Swedish Council on Health Technology Assessment, 2011); E. Sagen, *Transurethral Resection of the Prostate. Studies on Efficacy, Morbidity, and Costs* (academic dissertation, University of Gothenburg, 2020).

10. This is a term I borrow from Mol, *The Body Multiple*, to refer to the work of stabilizing different understandings and heterogeneous

practices, which makes an object (or a diagnosis) appear singular, unified, and uncontested. When bracketed, the ontological multiplicities appear singular. But the elements within the object or diagnosis also become largely invisible.

11. Or foreground it, as Mol would say.

12. American Urological Association, "Management of Benign Prostatic Hyperplasia"; Statens Beredning för Medicinsk och Social Utvärdering (SBU), *Godartad prostataförstoring med avflödeshinder*; J. de la Rosette et al., "Guidelines on Benign Prostatic Hyperplasia," European Association of Urology, 2006, https://uroweb.org/wp-content/uploads/EAU-Guidelines-BPH-2006.pdf; Foster et al., "Surgical Management of Lower Urinary Tract Symptoms," 7.

13. American Urological Association, "Management of Benign Prostatic Hyperplasia," 3.

14. SBU, *Godartad prostataförstoring med avflödeshinder*, 64.

15. "In the PSA era many men with BPH are identified because of having increased awareness of prostate cancer including the measurement of PSA as opposed to presenting primarily with bothersome lower urinary tract symptoms (LTS) as in the pre-PSA era." A. Sarma et al., "A Population Based Study of Incidence and Treatment of Benign Prostatic Hyperplasia Among Residents of Olmsted County, Minnesota: 1987–1997," *Journal of Urology* 173 (2005): 2048–2053. See also *Godartad prostataförstoring med avflödeshinder*.

16. American Urological Association, "Management of Benign Prostatic Hyperplasia," appendix, p. 280; see also Kellogg Parsons, "Modifiable Risk Factors for Benign Prostatic Hyperplasia," 395.

17. But it could have been otherwise, as STS scholars like to remind us. In medicine, we can trace how embodied experiences and practices become medical objects through a process of medicalization (see P. Conrad, *The Medicalization of Society: On the Transformation of Human Conditions into Treatable Disorders* [Baltimore: Johns Hopkins University Press, 2007]); J. Dumit, *Drugs for Life: How Pharmaceutical Companies Define Our Health* (Durham, NC: Duke University Press, 2012); R. Fox, "The Medicalization and Demedicalization of

American Society," *Daedalus* 106, no. 1 (1977); J. S. Williams et al., "The Pharmaceuticalization of Society? A Framework for Analysis," *Sociology of Health and Illness* 33, no. 5 (2011). Menstruation, pregnancy, and menopause are often-cited examples of healthy bodily functions which are now the object of medical care, as are aspects of mental health and sexuality. Pointing out a process of medicalization does not (necessarily) mean that becoming a medical object is unnecessary, but it does leave hanging in the air the possibility that some "problems" could be addressed in different ways.

18. S. Boyarsky et al., "A new look at bladder neck obstruction by the food and drug administration regulators: guide lines for investigation of benign prostatic hypertrophy." *Trans American Association of Genitourinology Surgery*, no. 68 (1976): 329–350.

19. These questions are used by the American Urological Association, which has endorsed, further developed, and spread them beyond their own membership to other professional bodies. For example, the European Association of Urology's guidelines on Benign Prostatic Hyperplasia recommend using what they call the International Prostate Symptom Score (I-PSS), with the same seven questions as above.

20. B. J. Hansen et al., "Validation of the Self-Administered Danish Prostatic Symptom Score (DAN-PSS-1) System for Use in Benign Prostatic Hyperplasia," *British Journal of Urology* 6, no. 4 (1995): 451–458; T. Peters et al., "The International Continence Society 'Benign Prostatic Hyperplasia' Study: The Bothersomeness of Urinary Symptoms," *The Journal of Urology* 157 (1997): 885–889.

21. H. A. Guess et al., "Similar Levels of Urological Symptoms have Similar Impact on Scottish and American Men—Although Scots Report Less Symptoms," *Journal of Urology* 150, no. 5, pt. 2 (1993): 1701–1705.

22. M. O'Leary, "Validity of the 'Bother Score' in the Evaluation and Treatment of Symptomatic Benign Prostatic Hyperplasia," *Review of Urology* 7, no. 1 (2005): 1–10.

23. Peters et al., "The Bothersomeness of Urinary Symptoms," 887.

24. O'Leary, "Validity of the 'Bother Score', Evaluation and Treatment," 1–10.

25. In the US, officially called the AUA Symptom Index for Benign Prostatic Hyperplasia (BPH) and the Disease Specific Quality of Life Question. See also Barry et al., "The American Urological Association Symptom Index for Benign Prostatic Hyperplasia," *Journal of Urology* 197, no. 25 (2017): S189–S197.

26. Foster et al., "Surgical Management of Lower Urinary Tract Symptoms," 612.

27. SBU, *Godartad prostataförstoring med avflödeshinder*, 283.

28. SBU, *Godartad prostataförstoring med avflödeshinder*, 284.

29. Two terms taken from Actor Network Theory; see B. Latour and S. Woolgar, *Laboratory Life: The Construction of Scientific Facts* (New York: Sage Publications, 1979). These numbers don't necessarily stay put in the patient's records, either. Data about ourselves moves and changes far beyond the original context of production; for this, see D. Lupton, *The Quantified Self: A Sociology of Self-Tracking* (Cambridge: Polity Press, 2016).

30. See Kellogg Parsons, "Modifiable Risk Factors for Benign Prostatic Hyperplasia," 395.

31. Here I would refer my graduate students back to Canguilhem's *On the Normal and the Pathological* (1978), but the rest of you can just keep reading.

32. C. J. Girman et al., "Natural History of Prostatism: Impact of Urinary Symptoms on Quality of life in 2,115 Randomly Selected Community Men," *Urology* 44, no. 6 (1994): 825–831.

33. S. J. Jacobsen et al., "A Population-Based Study of Health Care-Seeking Behavior for Treatment of Urinary Symptoms: The Olmsted County Study of Urinary Symptoms and Health Status Among Men," *Archives of Family Medicine* 2, no. 7 (1993): 730. For more details on this study, see also C. G. Chute et al., "The Prevalence of Prostatism: A Population-Based Survey of Urinary Symptoms," *Journal of Urology* 150, no. 1 (1993); S. J. Jacobsen et al., "Treatment for Benign Prostatic

Hyperplasia Among Community Dwelling Men: The Olmsted County Study of Urinary Symptoms and Health Status," *Journal of Urology*, 162, no. 4 (1999); Sarma et al., "A Population-Based Study of Incidence and Treatment"; de la Rosette et al., "Guidelines."

34. In a medical article reporting on the Olmsted County survey, Sarma et al. report that the residents of Olmsted County have good access to healthcare, are near a world-class provider (Mayo Clinic), and are mostly white, so "generalizing the incidence rates to persons of other races or settings may not be appropriate" (Sarma et al., "A Population-Based Study of Incidence and Treatment," 2053). I mention this to emphasize that it is not just critical social scientists who point out the potential problems with this.

35. American Urological Association, "Management of Benign Prostatic Hyperplasia," appendix, 2.

36. American Urological Association, "Management of Benign Prostatic Hyperplasia," appendix, 281.

37. Inscription practices, as Latour and Woolgar (1979) point out, are one of the practices in producing scientific facts from, among other things, laboratory work.

38. American Urological Association, "Management of Benign Prostatic Hyperplasia," appendix, 283.

39. M. Chancellor et al., "Bladder Outlet Obstruction versus Impaired Detrusor contractibility: The Role of Outflow," *Journal of Urology* 145, no. 4 (1991): 810–812.

40. American Urological Association, "Management of Benign Prostatic Hyperplasia," appendix, 283.

41. Here, again, I am taking a cue from Mol's (2002) work, and returning to the way knowledge is made through particular constellations of bodies, technologies, and practices.

42. American Urological Association, "Management of Benign Prostatic Hyperplasia," 280; SBU, *Godartad prostataförstoring med avflödeshinder*, 246.

43. SBU, *Godartad prostataförstoring med avflödeshinder*, 246.

44. In fact, there used to be an ongoing debate within the medical community about whether the GP's finger was better or worse than the urologist's finger when it comes to the DRE. See A-C. Kinn et al., *Prostata—mannens ständiga gissel* (Södertälje: Astra Sverige, 1997).

45. SBU, *Godartad prostataförstoring med avflödeshinder*, 246.

46. American Urological Association, "Management of Benign Prostatic Hyperplasia," 280; see also SBU, *Godartad prostataförstoring med avflödeshinder*, 245.

47. J. Winterich et al., "Masculinity and the Body: How African American and White Men Experience Cancer Screening Exams Involving the Rectum," *American Journal of Men's Health* 3, no. 4 (2009): 300–309.

48. For work on how these are taught in the USA, especially the gynecological exam, see K. Underman, *Feeling Medicine: How the Pelvic Exam Shapes Medical Training* (New York: New York University Press, 2020).

49. J. Gleisner and K. Siwe, "Differences in Teaching Female and Male Intimate Examinations: A Qualitative Study," *Medical Education* 54, no. 4 (2020): 348–355.

50. Gleisner and Siwe, "Differences in Teaching Female and Male Intimate Examinations."

51. J. Gleisner, "Prostataundersökningen och den (o)känslige mannen," in *Prostatan—det ständiga gisslet? Mannen och prostatan I kultur, medicin och historia*, ed. M. Björkman (Lund: Nordic Academic Press, 2018), 43–58.

52. G. Dowsett, "'Losing My Chestnut': One Gay Man's Wrangle with Prostate Cancer—Ten Years On," in *Gay and Bisexual Men Living with Prostate Cancer from Diagnosis to Recovery*, ed. J. M. Ussher, J. Perz, and B. R. S. Rosser (New York: Harrington Park Press, 2018), 264.

53. M. Bo et al., "Relationship between Prostatic Specific Antigen (PSA) and Volume of the Prostate in the Benign Prostatic Hyperplasia

in the Elderly," *Critical Reviews in Oncology/Hematology* 47, no. 3 (2003): 207–211.

54. K. Wailoo, *How Cancer Crossed the Color Line* (Oxford: Oxford University Press, 2011); for a history of its discovery and controversy, see H. K. Valier, *A History of Prostate Cancer: Cancer, Men and Medicine* (London: Palgrave Macmillan, 2016); for more on its controversy, see R. Ablin and R. Piana, *The Great Prostate Hoax: How Big Medicine Hijacked the PSA Test and Caused a Public Health Disaster* (New York: St. Martin's Press, 2014).

55. S. Jerak-Zuiderent, "A Feeling for Data—Screening and Researching Prostate Cancer with Care," in Björkman, ed., *Prostatan—det ständiga gisslet?*, 77–88.

56. Other medical tests work this way, too; for example, screening for cognitive decline or genetic screening for certain cancers; see S. Hesse-Biber, *Waiting for Cancer to Come: Women's Experiences with Genetic Testing and Medical Decision Making for Breast and Ovarian Cancer* (Ann Arbor: University of Michigan Press, 2014); K. Zeiler, "An Analytic Framework for Conceptualizations of Disease: Nine Structuring Questions and How Some Conceptualizations of Alzheimer's Disease Can Lead to Diseasisation," *Medicine, Health Care and Philosophy* 13, no. 4 (2020): 333–342.

57. S. Ciechanowski, *Prostatic Hypertrophy: Anatomical Researches on the So-Called "Prostatic Hypertrophy" and Allied Processes in the Bladder and Kidneys* (New York: Pelton, 1903), 12.

58. S. C. Martin, Jr., ed. *Prostatic Hypertrophy from Every Surgical Standpoint by George M. Phillips, M.D. and Forty Distinguished Authorities* (St. Louis: AJOD Company, Medical Publishers, 1903), 24.

59. Foster et al., "Surgical Management of Lower Urinary Tract Symptoms," 7.

60. In an agential realist framework, this would be called an onto-epistemological unit or a knowledge phenomenon; see K. Barad, *Meeting the Universe Halfway* (Durham: Duke University Press, 2007). It isn't necessarily a problem to make these cuts, and know the prostate as a thing. In fact, it is pretty necessary for the production of

prostate health within urology. But I hope I'm starting to show that it is also a material–discursive entanglement, and the cuts around it are to some degree arbitrary. Where we and urology make them is relevant to what further care can be provided.

61. Foster et al., "Surgical Management of Lower Urinary Tract Symptoms," 7.

62. B. Latour, *Science in Action: How to Follow Scientists and Engineers through Society* (Cambridge, MA: Harvard University Press, 1987).

63. What if, as a thought experiment, the object had been envisioned as the gland *and* the pelvic floor muscle? Or as a system also including the kidneys and bladder? How would this different understanding of the object, when combined with patient experiences of urination, produce different methods of diagnosis and treatment for LUTS? Instead of prescribing medication to change the prostate, or surgery to remove all or part of it, would treatments focus on pelvic floor muscle control, for example?

64. The alert reader may notice the allusion to E. Martin's *The Woman in the Body: A Cultural Analysis of Reproduction* (Boston: Beacon Press, 1987). More inspirational work about the relationship between bodies, expectations, politics, and medical knowledge can be found in B. Ehrenreich and D. English, *Witches, Midwives and Nurses: A History of Women Healers* (New York: Feminist Press at the City University of New York, 1973); A. Fausto-Sterling, *Sexing the Body: Gender Politics and the Construction of Sexuality* (New York: Basic Books, 2000); L. Jordanova, *Nature Displayed: Gender, Science and Medicine 1760–1820* (London: Longman, 1999); N. Oudshoorn, *Beyond the Natural Body* (London: Routledge, 1994); L. Schiebinger, *Nature's Body: Gender in the Making of Modern Science* (Boston: Beacon Press, 1993); C. Waldby, *The Visible Human Project: Informatic Bodies and Posthuman Medicine* (London: Routledge, 2000). For a discussion of the role activism has played in medical knowledge-making practices, see S. Epstein, *Inclusion: The Politics of Difference in Medical Research* (Chicago: University of Chicago Press, 2007); M. Murphy, *Seizing the Means of Reproduction: Entanglements of Feminism, Health and Technoscience* (Durham: Duke University Press, 2012); N. Tuana,

"The Speculum of Ignorance: The Women's Health Movement and Epistemologies of Ignorance," *Hypatia* 21, no. 3 (2006): 1–19; on how activism travels and is transformed, see K. Davis, *The Making of Our Bodies, Ourselves: How Feminism Travels Across Borders* (Durham: Duke University Press, 2007).

65. Mol, *The Body Multiple*; Barad, *Meeting the Universe Halfway*; E. Johnson, *Refracting through Technologies: Bodies, Medical Technologies and Norms* (London: Routledge, 2019).

66. There are so many interesting points to be made about how societies now (and historically) engage political understandings of bodies, categories, needs, and rights in the provision of public bathrooms. I would suggest beginning with some of these texts: S. Cavanagh, *Queering Bathrooms: Gender, Sexuality and the Hygienic Imagination* (Toronto: University of Toronto Press, 2010); P. A. Cooper and R. Oldenziel, "Cherished Classifications: Bathrooms and the Construction of Gender/Race on the Pennsylvania Railroad during World War II," *Feminist Studies* 25, no. 1 (1999): 7–41; O. Gershenson and B. Penner, *Ladies and Gents: Public Toilets and Gender* (Philadelphia: Temple University Press, 2009); G. Greed, "Public Toilet Provision for Women in Britain: An Investigation of Discrimination against Urination," *Women's Studies International Forum* 18, nos. 5/6 (1995): 573–584; B. Penner, *Bathroom* (London: Reaktion Books, 2014).

67. These sorts of solutions fall into the structural approach to disability studies, and also find traction with ideas in science and technology studies (see V. Galis, "We Have Never Been Able-Bodied: Thoughts on Dis/Ability and Subjectivity from Science and Technology Studies," in *Routledge Handbook of Disability Studies*, ed. Nick Watson and Simo Vihmas (London: Routledge, 2019); I. Moser, "A Body That Matters? The Role of Embodiment in the Recomposition of Life after a Road Traffic Accident," *Scandinavian Journal of Disability Research* 11, no. 2 (2009): 83–99; M. Schillmeier, *Rethinking Disability. Bodies, Senses and Things* (London: Routledge, 2010). Similar problems are addressed by the universal design field; see A. Hamraie, *Building Access: Universal Design and the Politics of Disability* (Minneapolis: University of Minnesota Press, 2017).

68. See Johnson, *Refracting through Technologies*.

Chapter 4

1. Some of these men found out about my study through social media or in social situations, or through a friend of a friend, and contacted *me*. On occasion, people just dropped by my office and told me I needed to know about their experience for my research. While I suspect this is very common in much social science research, it does turn ideas about following an intentional, predetermined study design, controlled subject selection, interview techniques (and ethics board reviews), and the power dynamics between interviewer and interviewee on their head. For discussions of this, see S. Hesse-Biber, "The Practice of Feminist In-Depth Interviewing," in *Feminist Research Practice: A Primer*, 2nd ed., ed. S. Nagy Hesse-Biber (Los Angeles: Sage Publishing, 2013), 111–138; C. Lundström, "White Ethnography: (Un)comfortable Conveniences and Shared Privileges in Field Work with Swedish Migrant Women," *NORA—Nordic Journal of Feminist and Gender Research* 18, no. 2 (2010): 70–87.

2. D. A. Leigh, "Prostatitis—An Increasing Clinical Problem for Diagnosis and Management," *Journal of Antimicrobial Chemotherapy* 32, suppl. A (1993): 1–9.

3. J. Krieger et al., "NIH Consensus Definition and Classification of Prostatitis," *Journal of the American Medical Association* 282, no. 3 (1999): 236–237; M. Giacomo et al., "Chronic Prostatitis: Current Treatment Options," *Research and Reports in Urology* 11 (2019): 165–174.

4. G. M. Habermacher et al., "Prostatitis/Chronic Pelvic Pain Syndrome," *Annual Review of Medicine* 57 (2006): 195–206; Giacomo et al., "Chronic Prostatitis."

5. E. Uustal, "Debatt: Nya strategier för behandling av långvarig bäckensmärta," *Läkartidningen*, https://lakartidningen.se/Opinion/Debatt/2016/12/Nya-strategier-for-behandling-av-langvarig-backensmarta/, accessed September 2020.

6.   B. Holmström and P. Hällberg, "Antibiotikabehandling vid kronisk prostatit saknar I princip evidens," *Läkartidningen* 48, no. 103
(2006): 3822–3828.

7.   A policy that has been framed as "rational use" in the Swedish
context, and pretty successful in reducing the number of prescrip-
tions written; see H. Gröndal, "The Emergence of Antimicrobial
Resistance as a Public Matter of Concern: A Swedish History of a
'Transformative Event'," *Science in Context* 31, no. 4 (2018): 477–500;
H. Gröndal, "Unpacking Rational Use of Antibiotics: Policy in Medical Practice and the Medical Debate," PhD diss., Uppsala University,
2018.

8.   M. Björkman and A. Persson, "What's in a Gland? Sexuality,
Reproduction, and the Prostate in Early-Twentieth-Century Medicine," *Gender and History* 32, no. 3 (2020): 621–636.

9.   W. Coutis and E. Silva-Inzunza, "Residual Prostatitis," *British
Medical Journal* (10 January 1948): 75.

10.   *British Medical Journal*, "Chronic Prostatitis" (1 July 1972). https://
www.bmj.com/content/bmj/3/5817/1.1.full.pdf

11.   *British Medical Journal*, "Chronic Prostatitis."

12.   *British Medical Journal*, "Chronic Prostatitis."

13.   Interview with a retired Swedish medical doctor.

14.   Gröndal, "The Emergence of Antimicrobial Resistance"; Gröndal,
"Unpacking Rational Use of Antibiotics."

15.   G. Perletti et al., "Antimicrobial Therapy for Chronic Bacterial
Prostatitis," *Cochrane Database of Systematic Reviews* 8, no. CD009071
(2013): 1.

16.   J. V. A. Franco et al., "Non-pharmacological Interventions
for Treating Chronic Prostatitis/Chronic Pelvic Pain Syndrome
(Review)," *Cochrane Database of Systematic Reviews* 5, no. CD012551
(2018): 3.

17.   Franco et al., "Non-pharmacological Interventions," 3.

18. Franco et al., "Non-pharmacological Interventions," 3.

19. *British Medical Journal*, "Chronic Prostatitis."

20. J. C. Gingell, "Chronic Prostatitis," *British Medical Journal* 295 (1987): 998.

21. Giacomo, "Chronic Prostatitis," 165; T. Parks, *Teach Us to Sit Still: A Sceptic's Search for Health and Healing* (London: Harvill Secker, 2001).

22. Gingell, "Chronic Prostatitis," 998.

23. https://docplayer.se/104681954-Backenbottensmarta-helena-hal lencreutz-grape-specialistsjukgymnast-uroterapeut-uroterapienheten -pf-benign-urologi-karolinska-universitetssjukhuset.html; https://www .sfog.se/media/336061/hela-baeckenbotten-anna-skawonius.pdf

24. I have translated *underliv* as "pelvic region." Literally, *underliv* means the anatomical volume beneath the belt, since *liv* is a word for a traditional piece of clothing that went around the waist, and this term referred to the area *under* it. While it often appears in gynecological discourses (and then usually as a trope for the internal reproductive organs), it can be equally applied to all bodies. The important aspect is the volumetric element; it means the space in the abdomen below the waist and everything that may be in it, including prostates.

25. See, for example, A. Swift, "Understanding Pain and the Human Body's Response to It," *Nursing Times* 114, no. 3 (2018): 22–26; L. McCracken and C. Eccleston, "Coping or Acceptance: What to Do about Chronic Pain?," *Pain* 105, nos. 1–2 (2003): 197–204; M. Wright et al., "Pain Acceptance, Hope, and Optimism: Relationships to Pain Adjustment in Patients with Chronic Musculoskeletal Pain," *Journal of Pain* 12, no. 11 (2011): 1155–1162. These ways of thinking about pain appear in both biomedical literature and work from within the medical humanities; see D. Leder, *The Absent Body* (Chicago: University of Chicago Press, 1990), and E. Scarry, *The Body in Pain* (Oxford: Oxford University Press, 1988). The discussion also touches on how some approaches theorize pain as a somatization of life (a difficult, stressful situation can manifest as pain), while others place pain as the element of study, itself, rather than trying to trace the source

to a life situation or a physical event or cause, thereby reproducing the dualism of mind/body (A. Kleinman, "Depression, Somatization and the 'New Cross-Cultural Psychiatry'," *Social Science and Medicine* 11, no. 1 [1977]: 3–10; L. J. Kirmayer, "Culture and the Metaphoric Mediation of Pain," *Transcultural Psychiatry* 45, no. 2 [2008]: 318–338). Talking about pain and admitting to it, the verbalization of how bad it is and what impact it has on daily life, is also affected by cultural expectations: M. S. Bates, "Ethnicity and Pain: A Biocultural Model," *Social Science and Medicine* 24, no. 1 (1987): 47–50; N. Mustafa et al., "The Lived Experiences of Chronic Pain among Immigrant Indian-Canadian Women: A Phenomenological Analysis," *Canadian Journal of Pain* 4, no. 3 (2020): 40–50; M. Perović et al., "Are You in Pain If You Say You Are Not: Accounts of Pain in Somali-Canadian Women With Female Genital Cutting (FGC)," *Pain* 162, no. 4 (2020): 1144–1152.

26. 1177 Vårdguiden. "Kronisk prostatit," healthcare counselling, online at https://www.1177.se/sjukdomar--besvar/konsorgan/prostata/k

27. See also E. Björk, "Att bota en prostata. Kastrering som behandlingsmetod för prostatahypertrofi 1893–1910," PhD diss., Linköping Studies in Arts and Sciences No. 774, Linköping University, 2019.

28. Wright et al., "Pain Acceptance, Hope, and Optimism"; M. Crowley-Matoka and G. True, "No-One Wants to be the Candy Man: Ambivalent Medicalization and Clinician Subjectivity in Pain Management," *Cultural Anthropology* 27, no. 4 (2012): 689–712; E. Vogel, "Restoring the Balance: Living Well with Pain," *Somatosphere: Science, Medicine and Anthropology*, http://somatosphere.net/2019/restoring-the-balance-living-well-with-pain.html/, 16 April 2019.

29. See 1177 Vårdguiden. "Kronisk prostatit."

30. For the analysis of how important visual media are to the production of breast cancer activist and advocacy communities, see L. Cartwright, "A Cultural Anatomy of the Visible Human Project," in *The Visible Woman: Imaging Technologies, Gender, and Science*, ed. P. Treichler et al. (New York: New York University Press, 1998), 21–43, and the discursive shifts that have occurred in breast cancer campaigns, particularly the reconfiguring of patients to survivors and the

adoption of a narrative of hope; see S. King, *Pink Ribbons Inc.: Breast Cancer and the Politics of Philanthropy* (Minneapolis: University of Minnesota Press, 2006).

31. Here the discussion of the inclusion and difference paradigm by S. Epstein in *Inclusion: The Politics of Difference in Medical Research* (Chicago: University of Chicago Press, 2007) is particularly relevant, but also his discussion of the way grass-roots activism has influenced scientific research; see S. Epstein, *Impure Science: AIDS, Activism, and the Politics of Knowledge* (Oakland: University of California Press, 1996).

32. Again, see K. Davis, "Feminist Body/Politics as World Traveller: Translating *Our Bodies, Ourselves*," *European Journal of Women's Studies* 9, no. 3 (2002): 223–247; M. Murphy, *Seizing the Means of Reproduction: Entanglements of Feminism, Health and Technoscience* (Durham: Duke University Press, 2012).

33. For a wonderful autobiographical description and reflection on this from a man's point of view, see Parks, *Teach Us to Sit Still*.

34. If you want to read more about this, start with D. Rosenfeld and C. Faircloth, eds., *Medicalized Masculinities* (Philadelphia: Temple University Press, 2006); B. Gough and S. Robertson, *Men, Masculinities and Health* (Basingstoke, UK: Palgrave Macmillan, 2010); and S. Robertson, *Understanding Men and Health: Masculinities, Identity and Well-Being* (Maidenhead, UK: Open University Press, 2007). Oliffe's work on masculinity and prostate cancer is also particularly relevant; see J. L. Oliffe, "Embodied Masculinity and Androgen Deprivation Therapy," *Sociology of Health and Illness* 28, no. 4 (2006): 410–432. Social norms of what it means to be a man become especially salient in discussions of reproduction; they have influenced the historical development of the fields of andrology and urology (see R. Almeling, *GUYnecology: The Missing Science of Men's Reproductive Health* [Oakland: University of California Press, 2020]; C. Bajeux, "Managing Masculinities: Doctors, Men, and Men's Partners Facing Male Infertility in France and French-speaking Switzerland (c.1890–1970)," *NORMA International Journal for Masculinity Studies* 15, no. 3 [2020]), and demonstrated the entanglement between sexuality and ageing

(see M. Loe, *The Rise of Viagra: How the Little Blue Pill Changed Sex in America* [New York: New York University Press, 2004]; B. Marshall, "'Hard Science': Gender Constructions of Sexual Dysfunction in the 'Viagra Age'," *Sexualities* 5, no. 2 [2002]: 141–158; B. Marshall, "The New Virility: Viagra, Male Aging and Sexual Function," *Sexualities* 9, no. 3 [2006]: 345–362; A. Potts, "Deleuze on Viagra (Or, What can a 'Viagra-Body' Do?)," *Body and Society* 10, no. 1 [2004]: 17–36; L. Sandberg, "Closer to Touch: Sexuality, Embodiment and Masculinity in Older Men's Lives," in *Ageing in Everyday Life: Materialities and Embodiments*, ed. S. Katz [Bristol, UK: Policy Press, 2018], 129–144; L. Tiefer, "The Viagra Phenomenon," *Sexualities* 9, no. 3 [2006]: 273–294).

35. See, on epistemologies of ignorance, N. Tuana, "The Speculum of Ignorance: The Women's Health Movement and Epistemologies of Ignorance," *Hypatia* 21, no. 3 (2006); and, specifically on men's reproductive health, Almeling, *GUYnecology*.

Chapter 5

1. It would take a book-length manuscript to properly describe the historical and current aspects of PSA controversies. Two which do this are H. K. Valier, "Screening, Patients, and the Politics of Prevention," in *A History of Prostate Cancer: Cancer, Men and Medicine* (London: Palgrave Macmillan, 2016); and R. Ablin and R. Piana, *The Great Prostate Hoax: How Big Medicine Hijacked the PSA Test and Caused a Public Health Disaster* (New York: St. Martin's Press, 2014).

2. Harvard Men's Health Watch, https://www.health.harvard.edu /newsletter_article/PSA-Prostate-Specific-Antigen-Persisting-Scientific -Ambiguities.

3. STHLM3 [Stockholm3 test], "About STHLM3," www.sthlm3.se, accessed September 2020.

4. S. Timmermans and M. Buchbinder, "Newborn Screening and Maternal Diagnosis: Rethinking Family Benefit," *Social Science and Medicine* 73, no. 7 (2011): 1014–1018; M. Gunnarson et al.,

"Ethico-Political Aspects of Conceptualising Screening: The Case of Dementia," *Health Care Analysis* (March 2021).

5.   O. Maldonado Castañeda, "Ett hälsosamt tillstånd av ovisshet. Tankar kring PSA-prov, förutsägbarhet och sårbarhet," in *Prostatan— det ständiga gisslet? Mannen och prostatan I kultur, medicin och historia*, ed. M. Björkman (Lund: Nordic Academic Press, 2018), 59–73.

6.   C. Kruse, "The Bayesian Approach to Forensic Evidence: Evaluating, Communicating, and Distributing Responsibility," *Social Studies of Science* 43, no. 5 (2012): 657–680.

7.   C. Gillespie, "The Experience of Risk as 'Measured Vulnerability': Health Screening and Lay Uses of Numerical Risk," *Sociology of Health and Illness* 34, no. 2 (2012): 194–207.

8.   Some can be found in S. Carlsson et al., "Anxiety Associated with Prostate Cancer Screening with Special Reference to Men with a Positive Screening Test (Elevated PSA): Results from a Prospective, Population-based, Randomised Study," *European Journal of Cancer* 43, no. 14 (2007): 2109–2116; R. C. Macefield et al., "Do the Risk Factors of Age, Family History of Prostate Cancer or a Higher Prostate Specific Antigen Level Raise Anxiety at Prostate Biopsy?," *European Journal of Cancer* 45, no. 14 (2009): 2569–2573; M-L. Essink-Bot et al., "Short-Term Effects of Population-Based Screening for Prostate Cancer on Health-Related Quality of Life," *Journal of the National Cancer Institute* 90, no. 12 (1998): 925–931.

9.   American Urological Association, "Early Detection of Prostate Cancer: AUA Guideline." American Urological Association, 2013.

10. R. Etzioni et al., "The Prostate Cancer Conundrum Revisited: Treatment Changes and Prostate Cancer Mortality Declines," *Cancer* 118, no. 23 (2012): 5955–5963.

11. J. L. Donovan et al., "Patient Reported Outcomes after Monitoring, Surgery, or Radiotherapy for Prostate Cancer," *New England Journal of Medicine* 375, no. 15 (2016): 1425–1437; R. Wassersug, "Getting Your PSA Checked Is Good for Overall Health," *Trends in Urology and Men's Health* (2016): 15.

12. T. Schlomm, "The Era of Prostate-Specific Antigen-Based Personalized Prostate Cancer Screening Has Only Just Begun," *European Urology* 68, no. 2 (2015): 2014–2015; M. A. Dall'Era et al., "Active Surveillance for Prostate Cancer: A Systematic Review of the Literature," *European Urology* 62, no. 6 (2012): 976–983; *Straits Times*, "Prostate Cancer Screening Better with New Thinking," https://www.straits times.com/singapore/health/prostate-cancer-screening-better-with -new-thinking, 5 October 2016.

13. For an example of activism around HIV/AIDS, see S. Epstein, *Impure Science: AIDS, Activism, and the Politics of Knowledge* (Oakland: University of California Press, 1996); for breast cancer, see M. Klawiter, *The Biopolitics of Breast Cancer: Changing Cultures of Disease and Activism* (Minneapolis: University of Minnesota Press, 2008).

14. For a literature review on prostate patient support groups, see L. Thaxton et al., "Prostate Cancer Support Groups," *Journal of Psychosocial Oncology* 23, no. 1 (2005): 25–40. Some of these support groups flourish, others don't; see J. L. Oliffe et al., "How Prostate Cancer Support Groups Do and Do Not Survive: British Columbian Perspectives," *American Journal of Men's Health* 2, no 2 (2008): 143–145. However, there is a difference between patient support groups and patient activism, even if those lines are sometimes blurred by the groups engaging in both.

15. D. Thorsén, "Epidemins aktörer. Patientkollektiv som maktfaktor: exemplet hiv/aids," *Socialmedicinsk tidskrift* 92, no. 6 (2016): 717–715; cf. Epstein, *Impure Science*; S. Epstein, *Inclusion: The Politics of Difference in Medical Research* (Chicago: University of Chicago Press, 2007); K. Wailoo et al., *Three Shots at Prevention: The HPV Vaccine and the Politics of Medicine's Simple Solutions* (Baltimore: Johns Hopkins University Press, 2010); J. Dunn et al., "Advocacy, Support and Survivorship in Prostate Cancer," *European Journal of Cancer Care* 27, no. 2 (2018): e12644.

16. P. C. Albertson, "The Prostate Cancer Conundrum," *Journal of the National Cancer Institute* 95, no. 13 (2003): 930–931; Etzioni et al., "The Prostate Cancer Conundrum Revisited"; N. Stone and E. Crawford, "To Screen or Not to Screen: The Prostate Cancer Dilemma,"

Asian Journal of Andrology 17, no. 1 (2015): 44–45; Socialstyrelsen, "Om PSA-prov. För att kunna upptäcka prostatacancer I ett tidigt skede—fördelar och nackdelar," Art. no. 2014-8-4 (2014): 1–6. https:// www.socialstyrelsen.se/globalassets/sharepoint-dokument/artikel katalog/kunskapsstod/2014-8-4.pdf; BBC, "Prostate Cancer Blood Test 'Helps Target Treatment'," 19 June 2017. http://www.bbc.com/news /health-40302692; DN 2017.

17. M. Annerstedt et al., "Agera Nu!" *Aftonbladet*, 1 February 2018, https://www.aftonbladet.se/debatt/a/ddm32J/agera-nu-innan-fler -dor-i-prostatacancer

18. R. Aschberg, "Prostatacancer vård. Var god, dröj." *Aftonbladet*, 5 February 2018, https://www.aftonbladet.se/nyheter/a/Qlx3wV/jag -slungades-in-i-en-varld-jag-inte-trodde-fanns

19. Mammography and breast cancer screening is often presented as an uncontroversial healthcare intervention, even though the scientific debate about its validity is not necessarily closed; see M. Kalager et al., "Effect of Screening Mammography on Breast-Cancer Mortality in Norway," *New England Journal of Medicine* 363, no. 13 (2010): 1203–1210.

20. L. Lindén, "Moving Evidence: Patient Groups, Biomedicine and Affects," *Science, Technology and Human Values* 35, no. 4 (2020): 444–473.

21. Socialstyrelsen, "Mer forskning om prostatacancerscreening behövs," https://www.socialstyrelsen.se/om-socialstyrelsen/pressrum /press/mer-forskning-om-prostatacancerscreening-behovs/, 12 February 2018; F. H. Schröder et al., "Screening and Prostate Cancer Mortality in a Randomized European Study," *New England Journal of Medicine* 360 (2009): 1320–1328; G. L. Andriole et al., "Mortality Results from a Randomized Prostate-Cancer Screening Trial," *New England Journal of Medicine* 360, no. 13 (2009): 1310–1319.

22. *Straits Times*, "Prostate Cancer Screening Better"; UK National Screening Committee, "The UK NSC Recommendation on Prostate Cancer Screening/PSA Testing in Men over the Age of 50," https:// legacyscreening.phe.org.uk/prostatecancer, January 2016.

23. P. Sakharkar and A. Kahaleh, "Age and Racial/Ethnic Disparities and Burden of Prostate Cancer: A Cross Sectional Population Based Study," *Journal of Basic and Clinical Pharmacy* 8 (2017): S022–S026.

24. R. J. Henderson et al., "Prostate-Specific Antigen (PSA) and PSA Density: Racial Differences in Men Without Prostate Cancer," *Journal of the National Cancer Institute* 89, no. 2 (1997): 134–138.

25. For a discussion of this in the medical literature, see R. Clegg et al., "Cancer Survival among U.S. Whites and Minorities: A SEER (Surveillance, Epidemiology and End Results) Program Population-Based Study," *Archives of Internal Medicine* 162, no. 17 (2002): 1985–1993; G. Hosain et al., "Racial/Ethnic Difference in Predictors of PSA Screening in a Tri-Ethnic Population," *Central European Journal of Public Health* 19, no. 1 (2011): 30–34. For a social science discussion, see K. Wailoo, *How Cancer Crossed the Colour Line* (Oxford: Oxford University Press, 2011), 156ff.

26. P. Finne et al., "Algorithms Based on Prostate-Specific Antigen (PSA), Free PSA, Digital Rectal Examination and Prostate Volume Reduce False-Positive PSA Results in Prostate Cancer Screening," *International Journal of Cancer* 111, no. 2 (2004): 310–315.

27. E. Johnson et al., *Glocal Pharma: International Brands and the Imagination of Local Masculinity* (London: Routledge, 2016); E. Johnson, *Refracting through Technologies: Bodies, Medical Technologies and Norms* (London: Routledge, 2019).

28. American Urological Association, "Early Detection of Prostate Cancer: AUA Guideline," American Urological Association, 2013; the UK National Screening Committee, "The UK NSC Recommendation"; 2016; the French Haute Autorité de Santé, "Cancer de la prostate: identification des facteurs de risque et pertinence d'un dépitage par dosage de l'antigène spécifique prostatique (PSA) de populations d'hommes à haut risque?," www.has-sante.fr, 4 April 2012; the National Cancer Centre Singapore, *Prostate Cancer.* https://www.nccs .com.sg/PatientCare/WhatisCancer/TypesofCancer/Pages/Prostate -Cancer.aspx, accessed September 2020.

29. GEKID, "Prostate," in *Cancer in Germany 2011/2012*, 10th ed. (Berlin: Prostate Cancer Zentrum für Krebsregisterdaten and Robert Koch Institut, 2012), https://www.krebsdaten.de/.

30. Socialstyrelsen, "Om PSA-prov. För att kunna upptäcka prostatacancer I ett tidigt skede—fördelar och nackdelar."

31. Svenska Dagbladet, "Skånska män erbjuds Prostataprov," https://www.svd.se/man-i-skane-erbjuds-prostataprov, *Svenska Dagbladet*, 26 June 2018.

32. M. Gunnarson et al., "Ethico-Political Aspects of Conceptualising Screening: The Case of Dementia," *Health Care Analysis* (March 2021).

33. For example, the classic, J. M. G. Wilson and G. Jungner, "Principles and Practice of Screening for Disease," Public Health Paper 34 (Geneva: World Health Organization, 1968).

34. N. Juth and C. Munthe, *The Ethics of Screening in Health Care and Medicine* (Heidelberg: Springer Verlag, 2012).

35. G. Edgren et al., "Screening, Case Finding or Primary Cancer Prevention in the Developing World?," *European Journal of Epidemiology* 28, no. 4 (2013): 287–290; Kalager et al., "Effect of Screening Mammography."

36. Schröder et al., "Screening and Prostate Cancer Mortality"; Andriole et al., "Mortality Results."

37. Two examples of lengthy academic texts which spend the necessary time to really delve into the nuances are Gunnarson et al., "Ethico-Political Aspects of Conceptualising Screening"; K. Zeiler and L. Käll, "Still Alice? Ethical Aspects of Conceptualising Selfhood in Dementia," in *The Routledge Handbook of the Medical Humanities*, ed. A. Bleakley (London: Routledge, 2020).

38. The report of the salon, in Swedish, can be found here: https://www.sverigesungaakademi.se/1454.html

39. Gunnarson et al., "Ethico-Political Aspects of Conceptualising Screening."

40. Medical humanities and STS work on healthcare does exactly the opposite. We try to articulate the complexity. The salon was an attempt to get these two different approaches to meet.

41. O. Maldonado Castañeda, "Price-Effectiveness: Pharmacoeconomics, Value and the Right Price for HPV Vaccines," *Journal of Cultural Economy* 10, no. 2 (2017): 163–177.

42. Maldonado Castañeda, "Ett hälsosamt tillstånd av ovisshet," 72.

43. Maldonado Castañeda, "Ett hälsosamt tillstånd av ovisshet," 72.

44. V. Adams et al., "Anticipation: Technoscience, Life, Affect, Temporality," *Subjectivity* 28, no. 1 (2009): 246–265; P. Maron, "Living Well with a Healthy Weight: A Case of the Body Mass Index as a Governing Practice," in manuscript.

Chapter 6

1. This is a topic discussed at length in phenomenology; see D. Leder, *The Absent Body* (Chicago: University of Chicago Press, 1990); K. Zeiler and L. Guntram "Sexed Embodiment in Atypical Pubertal Development: Intersubjectivity, Excorporation, and the Importance of Making Space for Difference," in *Feminist Phenomenology and Medicine*, ed. L. F. Käll and K. Zeiler (Albany, NY: SUNY Press, 2014), 141–160.

2. P. Cormie et al., "Improving Psychosocial Health in Men with Prostate Cancer through an Intervention that Reinforces Masculine Values—Exercise," *Psycho-Oncology* 25 (2016): 232–235; S. M. Rice et al., "Depression and Prostate Cancer: Examining Comorbidity and Male-Specific Symptoms," *American Journal of Men's Health* 12, no. 6 (2018): 1864–1872; J. M. Ussher, J. Perz, and B. R. S. Rosser, eds., *Gay and Bisexual Men Living with Prostate Cancer from Diagnosis to Recovery* (New York: Harrington Park Press 2018); C. Danemalm Jägervall and O. Bratt, *Sex, Samliv och Prostatacancer* (Växjö: Löwex Trycksaker AB (2019)).

3. See Leder, *The Absent Body*; K. Zeiler and L. F. Käll, "Still Alice? Ethical Aspects of Conceptualising Selfhood in Dementia," in

The Routledge Handbook of the Medical Humanities, ed. A. Bleakley (London: Routledge, 2014), 290–299.

4. For a longer discussion of this, see chapter 4 in E. Johnson, *Refracting through Technologies: Bodies, Medical Technologies and Norms* (London: Routledge, 2019).

5. Suggested reading for structural aspects of disability studies: V. Galis, "We Have Never Been Able-Bodied: Thoughts on Dis/Ability and Subjectivity from Science and Technology Studies," in *Routledge Handbook of Disability Studies*, ed. N. Watson and S. Vihmas (London: Routledge, 2019); I. Moser, "A Body That Matters? The Role of Embodiment in the Recomposition of Life after a Road Traffic Accident," *Scandinavian Journal of Disability Research* 11, no. 2 (2009): 83–99; M. Schillmeier, *Rethinking Disability. Bodies, Senses and Things.* (London: Routledge, 2010); and A. Hamraie, *Building Access: Universal Design and the Politics of Disability* (Minneapolis: University of Minnesota Press, 2017) on universal design.

6. When we started this work, we were keenly aware of the presumed heterosexuality in many of the conversations about prostate cancer, in discourse around it, and research about it (cf. J. Bergman and M. Litwin, "Foreword," in Ussher et al., *Gay and Bisexual Men*, ix). This can make prostate cancer rehabilitation even more painful for some men, who may feel marginalized by the way they are met in the clinical setting and by the heteronormative assumptions in the majority of information available to cancer patients (see Ussher et al., *Gay and Bisexual Men*, 18; G. Perlman, "Looking Back: Engaging Prostate Cancer as a Gay Man," in Ussher et al., *Gay and Bisexual Men*, 295; D. Doran et al., "It's Not Just about Prostate Cancer, It's about Being a Gay Man: A Qualitative Study of Gay Men's Experiences of Healthcare Provision in the UK," *European Journal of Cancer Care* 27, no. 6 [2018]). When one is confronted with even just the possibility of cancer, one is already in a vulnerable position, and may not have the strength or desire to also educate one's doctor or clinic that the presumptions of heterosexuality and a female partner are wrong. One may not feel like disclosing—and one is probably not even going to be asked about—one's sexuality or partners (see Ussher et al., *Gay and Bisexual Men*, 4). To address this silent heteronormativity, in addition to actually doing

research that integrated men who self-identify as gay within our projects, I am writing this section of the book as if results belonged to the global category "men," and when there appears, in the results or the literature, to be a difference between how gay men and heterosexual men experience an issue, I try to present the heterosexual experience as the modified and named category. With this I want to counteract the assumed heterosexual norm, but also acknowledge that all men's sexual practices are varied, and do not directly overlap with identity categories like hetero, gay, and bi.

7.   Some studies indicate that the loss of ejaculate (dry ejaculations) bothers heterosexual men less than gay and bisexual men; see B. R. S. Rosser, S. Hunt, B. Capistrant et al., "Understanding Prostate Cancer in Gay, Bisexual, and Other Men Who Have Sex with Men and Transgender Women," in Ussher et al., *Gay and Bisexual Men*, 2; Perlman, "Looking Back," in Ussher et al., *Gay and Bisexual Men*; C. Danemalm Jägervall, J. Brüggemann, and E. Johnson, "Gay Men's Experiences of Sexual Changes after Prostate Cancer Treatment—A Qualitative Study in Sweden," *Scandinavian Journal of Urology* 53, no. 1 (2019): 40–44.

8.   Ussher et al., *Gay and Bisexual Men*.

9.   For a very personal reflection on the side effects of prostate cancer treatments, see P. Steinberg, *A Salamander's Tale* (New York: Skyhorse, 2015).

10. Danemalm Jägervall and Bratt, *Sex, Samliv och Prostatacancer*.

11. Danemalm Jägervall and Bratt, *Sex, Samliv och Prostatacancer*.

12. See G. Dowsett, "'Losing My Chestnut': One Gay Man's Wrangle with Prostate Cancer—Ten Years On," in Ussher et al., *Gay and Bisexual Men*, 265.

13. Personal communication with C. Danemalm Jägervall, June 2020. This identification appears in much bi- and homosexual discourse, and Danemalm Jägervall and Jelmer Brüggemann note that their interview study with self-identifying gay men revealed anxiety about how anal penetration would be after prostatectomy (Danemalm Jägervall et al., "Gay Men's Experiences"). But some men who don't identify as gay also engage in prostate stimulation. Another

interesting contour of the prostate that appeared in the course of this project was the homology between the male prostate and the Skene's glands (and sometimes the G-spot, though this is slightly different). Without opening up another "is" about that part of the female anatomy, I am nonetheless fascinated by this discussion and the discursive power of that homology. When these two anatomical parts are paired, each gains from the other's legitimacy. The Skene's glands (and the G-spot, when that homology is made) can use the prostate's association with ejaculate and orgasm to legitimate its own relationship to female ejaculation. That is, after all, one of the primary functions of the male prostate—to help produce and pump out the ejaculate during orgasm. By associating itself with the prostate, the female ejaculation can legitimately claim the same practices. And the prostate can borrow the legitimacy of site-specific, intentional stimulation associated with, in particular, the G-spot. Think of all those women's magazine articles that describe in detail how to stimulate the G-spot for a modern, yet mainstream, readership. The prostate could benefit from that association, in an attempt to mainstream anal stimulation in sexual practices.

14. Danemalm Jägervall and Bratt, *Sex, Samliv och Prostatacancer.*

15. Danemalm Jägervall et al., "Gay Men's Experiences."

16. Danemalm Jägervall et al., "Gay Men's Experiences."

17. He uses the concept of repair work as it was developed by Persson (A. Persson, "An Unintended Side Effect of Pepper Spray: Gender Trouble and 'Repair Work' in an Armed Forces Unit," *Men and Masculinities* 15, no. 2 [2012]: 132–151) to address how an individual in a particular context reacts when something happens that disturbs their established way of doing gender (J. Brüggemann, "Redefining Masculinity—Men's Repair Work in the Aftermath of Prostate Cancer Treatment," *Health Sociology Review* 29, no. 3 [2020]: 5).

18. Brüggemann, "Redefining Masculinity."

19. This may be less true for men who self-identify as heterosexual (Brüggemann, "Redefining Masculinity"; see also T. K. Lee, A. B. Handy, W. Kwan, et al., "The Impact of Prostate Cancer Treatment

on the Sexual Quality of Life for Men-Who-Have-Sex-With-Men," *Journal of Sexual Medicine* 12, no. 2 [2015]: 2378–2386; S. Fry, "Perceptions of Prostate Cancer Risk in White Working Class, African Caribbean and Somali Men Living in South East Wales: A Constructivist Grounded Theory," PhD diss., Cardiff University, 2017; Ussher et al., *Gay and Bisexual Men*).

20. Heterosexual men may attend doctor appointments and treatment sessions alone less often than men in gay and bisexual relationships; see Doran et al., "It's Not Just about Prostate Cancer," 5–6.

21. Ussher et al., *Gay and Bisexual Men*.

22. K. Kenny et al., "Reciprocity, Autonomy, and Vulnerability in Men's Experiences of Informal Cancer Care," *Qualitative Health Research* 30, no. 4 (2019): 491–503.

23. Personal communication with Brüggemann, June 2020.

24. For a nuanced study of the motivations and experiences of leading prostate cancer support groups, see J. Dunn et al., "Advocacy, Support and Survivorship in Prostate Cancer," *European Journal of Cancer Care* 27, no. 2 (2018) e:12644.

25. Brüggemann, "Redefining Masculinity."

26. Dowsett, "'Losing My Chestnut'," 264.

27. V. Tangpricha and M. den Heijer, "Oestrogen and Anti-Androgen Therapy for Transgender Women," *The Lancet—Diabetes Endrocrinology* 5, no. 4 (2017): 291–300; R. Turo et al., "Metastatic Prostate Cancer in Transsexual Diagnosed after Three Decades of Estrogen Therapy," *Canadian Urology Association* 7, nos. 7–8 (2013); Ussher et al., *Gay and Bisexual Men*, 3; Rosser et al., "Understanding Prostate Cancer," in Ussher et al., *Gay and Bisexual Men*, 12.

28. M. Ingham et al., "Prostate Cancer in Transgender Women," *Urologic Oncology: Seminars and Original Investigations* 36, no. 12 (2018): 518–525; N. A. Deebel et al., "Prostate Cancer in Transgender Women: Incidence Etiopathogenesis, and Management Challenges," *Urology* 110 (2017): 166–171.

29. Thank you to T. Odland for this insight: personal communication, June 2020.

30. Danemalm Jägervall and Bratt, *Sex, Samliv och Prostatacancer*, 83. There is however, work that shows the rigidity of what is deemed an appropriate script for trans women to follow in conversations with medical authorities about their sexuality and their bodies (S. Bremer, "Penis at Risk: A Queer Phenomenology of Two Swedish Transgender Women's Narratives on Gender Correction," *Somatechnics* 3, no. 2 [2013]: 329–350), which should be considered. And on "the normative power of health (care) in the specific context of trans health (care)," see K. Harrison and U. Engdahl, "Guest Editors' Introduction," in "Trans Rights as Human Rights: The Implications for Trans Health (Care)," *Lambda Nordica* 18, nos. 3–4 (2013): 11. As I say in the main text, there is a lot more work to be done here.

31. Here, I think, there could be scope for generative conversations with trans studies literature on the idea of "real men" and "real women."

32. G. Einstein, "Situated Neuroscience: Elucidating a Biology of Diversity," in *Neurofeminism Issues at the Intersection of Feminist Theory and Cognitive Science*, ed. R. Bluhm, H. Maibom, and A. J. Jacobson (New York: Palgrave Macmillan 2012), 158.

33. This could be called decentering gender or an intersectional approach to health research; see O. Hankivsky, "Women's Health, Men's Health, and Gender and Health: Implications of Intersectionality," *Social Science and Medicine* 74, no. 11 (2012): 1712–1720.

Afterthoughts

1. D. Rosenfeld and C. Faircloth, eds., *Medicalized Masculinities* (Philadelphia: Temple University Press, 2006); B. Gough and S. Robertson, *Men, Masculinities and Health* (Basingstoke, UK: Palgrave Macmillan, 2010); S. Robertson, *Understanding Men and Health: Masculinities, Identity and Well-Being* (Maidenhead, UK: Open University Press, 2007); J. L. Oliffe, "Embodied Masculinity and Androgen Deprivation Therapy," *Sociology of Health and Illness* 28, no. 4 (2006):

410–432; I. Illich, *Limits to Medicine/Medical Nemesis: The Expropriation of Health* (London: Marion Boyars, 1975); E. Martin, *The Woman in the Body: A Cultural Analysis of Reproduction* (Boston: Beacon Press, 1987); A. Mol, *The Body Multiple* (Durham: Duke University Press, 2002); A. Fausto-Sterling, *Sexing the Body: Gender Politics and the Construction of Sexuality* (New York: Basic Books, 2000); L. Jordanova, *Nature Displayed: Gender, Science and Medicine 1760–1820* (London: Longman, 1999); N. Oudshoorn, *Beyond the Natural Body* (London: Routledge, 1994); M. Murphy, *Seizing the Means of Reproduction: Entanglements of Feminism, Health and Technoscience* (Durham: Duke University Press, 2012); N. Tuana, "The Speculum of Ignorance: The Women's Health Movement and Epistemologies of Ignorance," *Hypatia* 21, no. 3 (2006): 1–19; K. Davis, *The Making of Our Bodies, Ourselves: How Feminism Travels across Borders* (Durham: Duke University Press, 2007); D. Leder, *The Absent Body* (Chicago: University of Chicago Press, 1990); K. Zeiler, "A Phenomenological Analysis of Bodily Self-Awareness in the Experience of Pain and Pleasure: On Dys-Appearance and Eu-Appearance," *Medical Health Care and Philosophy* 13, no. 4 (2010): 333–342. See also the introduction of this volume.

2. For example, Martin, *The Woman in the Body*; B. Marshall, "The New Virility: Viagra, Male Aging and Sexual Function," *Sexualities* 9, no. 3 (2006): 345–362; K. Underman, *Feeling Medicine: How the Pelvic Exam Shapes Medical Training* (New York: New York University Press, 2020).

3. Davis, *The Making of Our Bodies, Ourselves*; Murphy, *Seizing the Means of Reproduction*; S. Epstein, *Inclusion: The Politics of Difference in Medical Research* (Chicago: University of Chicago Press, 2007).

4. S. Epstein, *Impure Science: AIDS, Activism, and the Politics of Knowledge* (Oakland: University of California Press, 1996); Murphy, *Seizing the Means of Reproduction*.

Bibliography

1177 Vårdguiden. "Kronisk prostatit." Healthcare counseling, online at https://www.1177.se/sjukdomar--besvar/konsorgan/prostata/kronisk -prostatit/

Ablin, R., and R. Piana. *The Great Prostate Hoax: How Big Medicine Hijacked the PSA Test and Caused a Public Health Disaster.* New York: St. Martin's Press, 2014.

Adams, V., M. Murphy, and A. E. Clarke. "Anticipation: Technoscience, Life, Affect, Temporality." *Subjectivity* 28, no. 1 (2009): 246–265.

Albertson, P. C. "The Prostate Cancer Conundrum." *Journal of the National Cancer Institute* 95, no. 13 (2003): 930–931.

Almeling, R. *GUYnecology: The Missing Science of Men's Reproductive Health.* Oakland: University of California Press, 2020.

American Urological Association. "American Urological Association Guideline: Management of Benign Prostatic Hyperplasia (BPH). (Revised)." Linthicum, MD: American Urological Association, 2010.

American Urological Association. "Early Detection of Prostate Cancer: AUA Guideline." Linthicum, MD: American Urological Association, 2013.

Anderson, W. "A Case of Chronic Prostatitis: A Pathological Contribution to the Study of the Physiology of the Prostate Gland." *British Medical Journal* (July 1887): 237.

Anderson, W. "Chronic Prostatitis and Aspermatism." *British Medical Journal* (August 1887): 483.

Andriole, G. L., E. D. Crawford, R. L. Grubb III., et al. "Mortality Results from a Randomized Prostate-Cancer Screening Trial." *New England Journal of Medicine* 360, no. 13 (2009): 1310–1319.

Annerstedt, M., K. Enhager, L. Falkman, et al. "Agera Nu!" *Aftonbladet*, 1 February 2018. https://www.aftonbladet.se/debatt/a/ddm32J /agera-nu-innan-fler-dor-i-prostatacancer

Appadurai, A., ed. *The Social Life of Things: Commodities in Cultural Perspective*. New York: Cambridge University Press, 1986.

Arnaud, S. *On Hysteria. The Invention of a Medical Category between 1670 and 1820*. Chicago: University of Chicago Press, 2015.

Åsberg, C., and E. Johnson. "Viagra Selfhood: Pharmaceutical Advertising and the Visual Formations of Swedish Masculinity." In *Glocal Pharma: International Brands and the Imagination of Local Masculinity* by E. Johnson, with E. Sjögren and C. Åsberg, 88–98. London: Routledge, 2016.

Aschberg, R. "Prostatacancer vård. Var god, dröj." *Aftonbladet*, 5 February 2018. https://www.aftonbladet.se/nyheter/a/Qlx3wV/jag-slun gades-in-i-en-varld-jag-inte-trodde-fanns

Bajeux, C. "Managing Masculinities. Doctors, Men, and Men's Partners Facing Male Infertility in France and French-Speaking Switzerland (c.1890–1970)." *NORMA: International Journal for Masculinity Studies* 15, no. 3 (2020). https://doi.org/10.1080/18902138.2020.180 5887

Balint, M. *The Doctor, His Patient and the Illness*. London: Pitman, 1957.

Barad, K. *Meeting the Universe Halfway*. Durham: Duke University Press, 2007.

Barry, M. J., F. J. Fowler, M. P. O'Leary, R. C. Bruskewitz, H. L. Holtgrewe, W. K. Mebust, A. T. Cockett, et al. "The American Urological

Association Symptom Index for Benign Prostatic Hyperplasia." *Journal of Urology* 197, no. 25 (February 2017): S189–S197.

Bates, M. S. "Ethnicity and Pain: A Biocultural Model." *Social Science and Medicine* 24, no. 1 (1987): 47–50.

BBC. "Prostate Cancer Blood Test 'Helps Target Treatment'." 19 June 2017. http://www.bbc.com/news/health-40302692

Becker, H. S., B. Geer, E. C. Hughes, and A. L. Strauss. *Boys in White: Student Culture in Medical School.* New Brunswick, NJ: Transaction Publishers, 1961.

Benninghaus, C. "Beyond Constructivism? Gender, Medicine and the Early History of Sperm Analysis, Germany 1870–1900." *Gender and History* 24 (2012): 647–676.

Bergman, J., and M. Litwin. "Foreword." In *Gay and Bisexual Men Living with Prostate Cancer from Diagnosis to Recovery,* edited by J. M. Ussher, J. Perz, and B. R. S. Rosser, ix–x. New York: Harrington Park Press, 2018.

Björk, E. "Att bota en prostata. Kastrering som behandlingsmetod för prostatahypertrofi 1893–1910." PhD diss., Linköping Studies in Arts and Sciences No. 774. Linköping University, 2019.

Björkman, M., ed., *Prostatan—det ständiga gisslet? Mannen och prostatan I kultur, medicin och historia.* Lund: Nordic Academic Press, 2018.

Björkman, M., and A. Persson. "What's in a Gland? Sexuality, Reproduction and the Prostate in Early Twentieth-Century Medicine." *Gender and History* 32, no. 3 (2020): 621–636.

Bo, M., M. Ventura, R. Marinello, S. Capello, G. Casetta, and F. Fabris. "Relationship between Prostatic Specific Antigen (PSA) and Volume of the Prostate in the Benign Prostatic Hyperplasia in the Elderly." *Critical Reviews in Oncology/Hematology* 47, no. 3 (2003): 207–211.

Boyarsky, S., G. Jones, D. F. Paulson, and G. R. Prout Jr. "A New Look at Bladder Neck Obstruction by the Food and Drug Administration Regulators: Guide Lines for Investigation of Benign Prostatic

Hypertrophy." *Trans American Association of Genitourinology Surgery*, no. 68(1976): 329–350.

Bremer, S. "Penis as Risk: A Queer Phenomenology of Two Swedish Transgender Women's Narratives on Gender Correction." *Somatechnics* 3, no. 2 (2013): 329–350.

British Medical Journal. "Chronic Prostatitis." 1 July 1972. https://www.bmj.com/content/bmj/3/5817/1.1.full.pdf

Brüggemann, J. "Redefining Masculinity—Men's Repair Work in the Aftermath of Prostate Cancer Treatment." *Health Sociology Review* 29, no. 3 (2020). https://doi.org/10.1080/14461242.2020.1820367

Burrell, S., and G. Gill. "The Liverpool Cholera Epidemic of 1832 and Anatomical Dissection—Medical Mistrust and Civil Unrest." *Journal of the History of Medicine and Allied Sciences* 60, no. 4 (2005): 478–498.

Canguilhem, G. *On the Normal and the Pathological*. London: Kluwer Academic Publishers, 1978.

Carlsson, S., G. Aus, C. Wessman, and H. Hugosson. "Anxiety Associated with Prostate Cancer Screening with Special Reference to Men with a Positive Screening Test (Elevated PSA): Results from a Prospective, Population-based, Randomised Study." *European Journal of Cancer* 43, no. 14 (2007): 2109–2116.

Cartwright, L. "A Cultural Anatomy of the Visible Human Project." In *The Visible Woman: Imaging Technologies, Gender, and Science*, edited by P. Treichler, L. Cartwright, and C. Penley, 21–43. New York: New York University Press, 1998.

Cavanagh, S. *Queering Bathrooms: Gender, Sexuality and the Hygienic Imagination*. Toronto: University of Toronto Press, 2010.

Chute, C. G., L. A. Panser, C. J. Girman, J. E. Oesterling, H. A. Guess, S. J. Jacobsen, and M. M. Lieber. "The Prevalence of Prostatism: A Population-Based Survey of Urinary Symptoms." *Journal of Urology* 150, no. 1 (1993): 85–89.

Ciechanowski, S. *Prostatic Hypertrophy: Anatomical Researches on the So-Called "Prostatic Hypertrophy" and Allied Processes in the Bladder and Kidneys*. New York: Pelton, 1903.

Clegg, L., F. Li, B. Hankey, K. Chu, and B. Edwards. "Cancer Survival among U.S. Whites and Minorities: A SEER (Surveillance, Epidemiology and End Results) Program Population-Based Study." *Archives of Internal Medicine* 162, no. 17 (2002): 1985–1993.

Conrad, P. *The Medicalization of Society: On the Transformation of Human Conditions into Treatable Disorders*. Baltimore: Johns Hopkins University Press, 2007.

Cooper, P. A., and R. Oldenziel. "Cherished Classifications: Bathrooms and the Construction of Gender/Race on the Pennsylvania Railroad during World War II." *Feminist Studies* 25, no. 1 (1999): 7–41.

Cormie, P., J. L. Oliffe, A. C. Wootten, D. A. Galvao, R. U. Newton, and S. K. Chambers. "Improving Psychosocial Health in Men with Prostate Cancer through an Intervention that Reinforces Masculine Values—Exercise." *Psycho-Oncology* 25 (2016): 232–235.

Coser, R. L. "Alienation and the Social Structure: Case Analysis of a Hospital." In *The Hospital in Modern Society: Eleven Stories of the Hospital Today*, edited by E. Freidson. London: Free Press of Glencoe, 1963.

Coutis, W., and E. Silva-Inzunza. "Residual Prostatitis." *British Medical Journal* (10 January 1948): 75.

Crowley-Matoka, M., and G. True. "No One Wants to Be the Candy Man: Ambivalent Medicalization and Clinician Subjectivity in Pain Management." *Cultural Anthropology* 27, no. 4 (2012): 689–712.

Dall'Era, M. A., P. C. Albertsen, C. Bangma, P. R. Carroll, H. B. Carter, et al. "Active Surveillance for Prostate Cancer: A Systematic Review of the Literature." *European Urology* 62, no. 6 (2012): 976–983.

Danemalm Jägervall, C., and O. Bratt. *Sex, Samliv och Prostatacancer*. Växjö: Löwex Trycksaker AB, 2019. https://prostatacancerforbundet.reklamlogistik.se/sv/informationsmaterial/bok-sex-samliv-prostatacancer.html

Danemalm Jägervall, C., J. Brüggemann, and E. Johnson. "Gay Men's Experiences of Sexual Changes after Prostate Cancer Treatment—A Qualitative Study in Sweden." *Scandinavian Journal of Urology* 53, no. 1 (2019): 40–44.

Daston, L. *Biographies of Scientific Objects*. Chicago: University of Chicago Press, 2000.

Davis, K. "Feminist Body/Politics as World Traveller: Translating *Our Bodies, Ourselves*." *European Journal of Women's Studies* 9, no. 3 (2002): 223–247.

Davis, K. *The Making of* Our Bodies, Ourselves: *How Feminism Travels Across Borders*. Durham: Duke University Press, 2007.

Deebel, N. A., J. P. Morin, R. Autorino, R. Vince, B. Grob, and L. J. Hampton. "Prostate Cancer in Transgender Women: Incidence, Etiopathogenesis, and Management Challenges." *Urology* 110 (2017): 166–171. https://doi.org/10.1016/j.urology.2017.08.032

de la Rosette, J., G. Alivizatos, S. Madersbacher, C. Rioja Sanz, J. Nordling, M. Emberton, S. Gravas, M. C. Michel, and M. Oelke. "Guidelines on Benign Prostatic Hyperplasia." European Association of Urology, 2006. https://uroweb.org/wp-content/uploads/EAU-Guidelines-BPH-2006.pdf

DN Debatt. "Dags för allmän screening för att hitta prostatacancer." *Dagensnyheter*, 2 April 2017.

Donovan, J. L., F. C. Hamdy, J. Athene Lane, et al. "Patient Reported Outcomes after Monitoring, Surgery, or Radiotherapy for Prostate Cancer." *New England Journal of Medicine* 375, no. 15 (2016): 1425–1437.

Doran, D., S. Williamson, M. Wright, and K. Beaver. "'It's Not Just about Prostate Cancer, It's About Being a Gay Man': A Qualitative Study of Gay Men's Experiences of Healthcare Provision in the UK." *European Journal of Cancer Care* 27, no. 6 (2018): e12923.

Dowsett, G. "'Losing My Chestnut': One Gay Man's Wrangle with Prostate Cancer—Ten Years On." In *Gay and Bisexual Men Living with Prostate Cancer from Diagnosis to Recovery*, edited by J. M. Ussher, J. Perz, and B. R. S. Rosser, 258–270. New York: Harrington Park Press, 2018.

Dumit, J. *Drugs for Life: How Pharmaceutical Companies Define Our Health*. Durham: Duke University Press, 2012.

Dunn, J., C. Casey, D. Dandoe, M. Hyde, M-C. Cheron-Sauer, A. Lowe, J. Oliffe, and S. Chambers. "Advocacy, Support and Survivorship in Prostate Cancer." *European Journal of Cancer Care* 27, no. 2 (2018): e12644.

Eaton, J., and R. Weil. *Culture and Mental Disorders.* Glencoe, IL: Free Press, 1955.

Edgren, G., P. Lagiou, D. Trichopoulos, and H-O. Adami. "Screening, Case Finding or Primary Cancer Prevention in the Developing World?" *European Journal of Epidemiology* 28, no. 4 (2013): 287–290.

Ehrenreich, B., and D. English, *Witches, Midwives and Nurses: A History of Women Healers.* New York: Feminist Press at the City University of New York, 1973.

Einstein, G. "Situated Neuroscience: Elucidating a Biology of Diversity." In *Neurofeminism: Issues at the Intersection of Feminist Theory and Cognitive Science,* edited by R. Bluhm, H. Maibom, and A. J. Jacobson, 145–174. New York: Palgrave Macmillan, 2012.

Einstein, G., A. S. Au, J. Klemensberg, E. M. Shin, and N. Pun. "The Gendered Ovary: Whole Body Effects of Oophorectomy." *Canadian Journal of Nursing Research* 44, no. 3 (2012): 7–17.

Epstein, S. *Impure Science: AIDS, Activism, and the Politics of Knowledge.* Oakland: University of California Press, 1996.

Epstein, S. *Inclusion: The Politics of Difference in Medical Research.* Chicago: University of Chicago Press, 2007.

Epstein, S. "Sex Differences and the New Politics of Women's Health." In *Inclusion: The Politics of Difference in Medical Research,* 233–257. Chicago: University of Chicago Press, 2007.

Essink-Bot, M-L., H. J. de Koning, H. G. Nijs, W. J. Kirkels, P. J. van der Maas, and F. H. Schröder. "Short-Term Effects of Population-Based Screening for Prostate Cancer on Health-Related Quality of Life." *Journal of the National Cancer Institute* 90, no. 12 (1998): 925–931.

Etzioni, R., R. Gulati, A. Tsodikov, E. M. Wever, et al. "The Prostate Cancer Conundrum Revisited: Treatment Changes and Prostate Cancer Mortality Declines." *Cancer* 118, no. 23 (2012): 5955–5963.

Fall, M. "Urininkontinens hos mannen—ett försummat problem?" *Läkartidningen* 96, no. 18 (1999): 2227–2231.

Fausto-Sterling, A. *Sexing the Body: Gender Politics and the Construction of Sexuality*. New York: Basic Books, 2000.

Finne P., R. Finne, C. Bangma, J. Hugosson, M. Hakama, A. Auvinen, and U. H. Stenman. "Algorithms Based on Prostate-Specific Antigen (PSA), Free PSA, Digital Rectal Examination and Prostate Volume Reduce False-Positive PSA Results in Prostate Cancer Screening." *International Journal of Cancer* 111, no. 2 (2004): 310–315.

Fleck, L. "The Problem of Epistemology" (1936). In *Cognition and Fact: Materials on Ludwik Fleck*, edited by R. S. Cohen and T. Schnelle. Boston Studies in the Philosophy of Science. Dordrecht: Reidel, 1986.

Foster, H., M. Barry, P. Dahm, M. Gandhi, S. Kaplan, T. Kohler, L. Lerner, D. Lightner, J. Kellogg Parsons, C. Roehrborn, C. Welliver, T. Wilt, and K. McVary. "Surgical Management of Lower Urinary Tract Symptoms Attributed to Benign Prostatic Hyperplasia. AUA Guideline." Linthicum, MD: American Urological Association, 2019.

Fox, R. *Experiment Perilous: Physicians and Patients Facing the Unknown*. Glencoe, IL: Free Press, 1959.

Fox, R. "The Medicalization and Demedicalization of American Society." *Daedalus* 106, no. 1 (1977): 9–22.

Frampton, S. *Belly-Rippers, Surgical Innovation and the Ovariotomy Controversy*. London: Palgrave Macmillan, 2018.

Franco, J. V. A., T. Turk, J. H. Jung, Y. T. Xiao, S. Iakhno, V. Garrote, and V. Vietto. "Non-Pharmacological Interventions for Treating Chronic Prostatitis/Chronic Pelvic Pain Syndrome (Review)." *Cochrane Database of Systematic Reviews* 5, no. CD012551 (2018).

Freidson, E. *The Hospital in Modern Society: Eleven Stories of the Hospital Today*. London: Free Press of Glencoe, 1963.

Friedrich, K. "From 'Imaging 2.0' to 'Imaging 3.0'." In *Scientific Knowledge and the Transgression of Boundaries*, edited by B-J. Krings, H.

Rodríguez, and A. Schleisiek, 35–57. Berlin: Verlag für Sozialwissenschaften, 2016.

Fry, S. "Perceptions of Prostate Cancer Risk in White Working Class, African Caribbean and Somali Men Living in South East Wales: A Constructivist Grounded Theory." PhD dissertation, Cardiff University, 2017.

Galis, V. "We Have Never Been Able-Bodied: Thoughts on Dis/Ability and Subjectivity from Science and Technology Studies." In *Routledge Handbook of Disability Studies*, edited by N. Watson and S. Vihmas, 404–418. London: Routledge, 2019.

GEKID. "Prostate." In *Cancer in Germany 2011/2012*, 10th ed., 94–97. Berlin: Prostate Cancer Zentrum für Krebsregisterdaten and Robert Koch Institut, 2012. https://www.krebsdaten.de/

Gershenson, O., and B. Penner. *Ladies and Gents: Public Toilets and Gender*. Philadelphia: Temple University Press, 2009.

Giacomo, M., T. Verdacchi, S. Rosadi, F. Annino, and M. De Angelis. "Chronic Prostatitis: Current Treatment Options." *Research and Reports in Urology* 11 (2019): 165–174.

Gilbert, S., and S. Gubar. *The Madwoman in the Attic: The Woman Writer and the Nineteenth-Century Literary Imagination*. New Haven: Yale University Press, 1979.

Gillespie, C. "The Experience of Risk as 'Measured Vulnerability': Health Screening and Lay Uses of Numerical Risk." *Sociology of Health and Illness* 34, no. 2 (2012): 194–207.

Gingell, J. C. "Chronic Prostatitis." *British Medical Journal* 295 (17 October 1987): 998.

Girman, C. J., R. Epstein, S. Jacobsen, H. Guess, L. Panser, J. Oesterling, and M. Lieber. "Natural History of Prostatism: Impact of Urinary Symptoms on Quality of Life in 2,115 Randomly Selected Community Men." *Urology* 44, no. 6 (1994): 825–831.

Gleisner, J. "Prostataundersökningen och den (o)känslige mannen." In *Prostatan—det ständiga gisslet? Mannen och prostatan I kultur, medicin och historia*, edited by M. Björkman, 43–58. Lund: Nordic Academic Press, 2018.

Gleisner, J., and K. Siwe. "Differences in Teaching Female and Male Intimate Examinations: A Qualitative Study." *Medical Education* 54, no. 4 (2020): 348–355.

Goddard, J. "The Prostate in Five Pictures." *Journal of Clinical Urology* 12, no. 15 (2019): 4–8.

Gosden, C., and Y. Marshall. "The Cultural Biography of Objects." *World Archaeology* 31, no. 2 (1999): 169–178.

Gough, B., and S. Robertson. *Men, Masculinities and Health: Critical Perspectives*. Basingstoke, UK: Palgrave Macmillan, 2010.

Greed, C. "Public Toilet Provision for Women in Britain. An Investigation of Discrimination Against Urination." *Women's Studies International Forum* 18, nos. 5/6 (1995): 573–584.

Gröndal, H. "The Emergence of Antimicrobial Resistance as a Public Matter of Concern: A Swedish History of a 'Transformative Event'." *Science in Context* 31, no. 4 (2018): 477–500.

Gröndal, H. "Unpacking Rational Use of Antibiotics: Policy in Medical Practice and the Medical Debate." PhD dissertation, Uppsala University, 2018.

Guess, H. A., C. Chute, W. Garraway, G. Girman, P. Panswer, R. Lee, S. Jacobsen, G. McKelvie, J. Oesterling, and M. Lieber. "Similar Levels of Urological Symptoms have Similar Impact on Scottish and American Men—Although Scots Report Less Symptoms." *Journal of Urology* 150, no. 5, pt. 2 (1993): 1701–1705.

Gunnarson, M., A. Kapeller, and K. Zeiler. "Ethico-Political Aspects of Conceptualising Screening: The Case of Dementia." *Health Care Analysis* (March 2021).

Habermacher, G. M., J. T. Chason, and A. J Schaeffer. "Prostatitis/ Chronic Pelvic Pain Syndrome." *Annual Review of Medicine* 57 (2006): 195–206.

Hamraie, A. *Building Access: Universal Design and the Politics of Disability.* Minneapolis: University of Minnesota Press, 2017.

Hankivsky, O. "Women's Health, Men's Health, and Gender and Health: Implications of Intersectionality." *Social Science and Medicine* 74, no. 11 (2012): 1712–1720.

Hansen, B. J., H. Flyger, K. Brasso, J. Schou, J. Nordling, J. Thorup Andersen, S. Mortensen, H. Meyoff, S. Walter, and T. Hald. "Validation of the Self-Administered Danish Prostatic Symptom Score (DAN-PSS-1) System for Use in Benign Prostatic Hyperplasia." *British Journal of Urology* 76, no. 4 (1995): 451–458.

Haraway, D. J. *Modest_Witness@Second_Millennium. FemaleMan©_ Meets_OncoMouse™: Feminism and Technoscience.* New York: Routledge, 1997.

Harrison, K., and U. Engdahl. "Guest Editors' Introduction." In "Trans Rights as Human Rights: The Implications for Trans Health (Care)." *Lambda Nordica* 18, nos. 3–4 (2013): 10–28.

Harvard Men's Health Watch. "PSA: Prostate-Specific Antigen, Persisting Scientific Ambiguities." https://www.health.harvard.edu/news letter_article/PSA-Prostate-Specific-Antigen-Persisting-Scientific-Ambi guities, July 2009.

Haute Autorité de Santé. "Cancer de la prostate: identification des facteurs de risque et pertinence d'un dépistage par dosage de l'antigène spécifique prostatique (PSA) de populations d'hommes à haut risque?" www.has-sante.fr, 4 April 2012.

Henderson, R. "What about Me?" In *Gay and Bisexual Men Living with Prostate Cancer from Diagnosis to Recovery,* edited by J. M. Ussher, J. Perz, and B. R. S. Rosser, 272–282. New York: Harrington Park Press.

Henderson, R. J., J. A. Eastham, D. J. Culkin, M. Kattan, T. Whatley, J. Mata, D. Venable, and O. Sartor. "Prostate-Specific Antigen (PSA) and PSA Density: Racial Differences in Men Without Prostate Cancer." *Journal of the National Cancer Institute* 89, no. 2 (1997): 134–138.

Hesse-Biber, S. "The Practice of Feminist In-Depth Interviewing." In *Feminist Research Practice: A Primer*, 2nd ed., edited by S. Nagy Hesse-Biber, 111–138. Los Angeles: Sage Publishing, 2013.

Hesse-Biber, S. *Waiting for Cancer to Come: Women's Experiences with Genetic Testing and Medical Decision Making for Breast and Ovarian Cancer.* Ann Arbor: University of Michigan Press, 2014.

Heyns, C. F., and D. P. de Klerk. "Pharmaceutical Management of Benign Prostatic Hyperplasia." In *Notes from Prostatic Disorders*, edited by D. Paulson, 204–231. London: Lea & Febiger, 1989.

Holmström, B., and P. Hällberg. "Antibiotikabehandling vid kronisk prostatit saknar I princip evidens." *Läkartidningen* 48, no. 103 (2006): 3822–3828.

Hosain, G., M. Sanderson, X. Du, W. Chan, and S. Strom. "Racial/Ethnic Difference in Predictors of PSA Screening in a Tri-Ethnic Population." *Central European Journal of Public Health* 19, no. 1 (2011): 30–34.

Hoskins, J. *Biographical Objects: How Things Tell the Story of People's Lives.* London: Routledge, 1998.

Illich, I. *Limits to Medicine/Medical Nemesis: The Expropriation of Health.* London: Marion Boyars, 1975.

Ingham, M., R. Lee, D. MacDermed, and A. Olumi. "Prostate Cancer in Transgender Women." *Urologic Oncology: Seminars and Original Investigations* 36, no. 12 (2018): 518–525.

Jacobsen, S. J., H. A. Guess, L. Panser, C. J. Girman, C. G. Chute, J. E. Oesterling, and M. M. Lieber. "A Population-Based Study of Health Care-Seeking Behavior for Treatment of Urinary Symptoms: The Olmsted County Study of Urinary Symptoms and Health Status among Men." *Archives of Family Medicine* 2, no. 7 (1993): 729–735.

Jacobsen, S. J., D. J. Jacobson, C. J. Girman, R. O. Roberts, T. Rhodes, H. A. Guess, and M. M. Lieber. "Treatment for Benign Prostatic Hyperplasia among Community Dwelling Men: The Olmsted County Study of Urinary Symptoms and Health Status." *Journal of Urology* 162, no. 4 (1999): 1301–1306.

Jerak-Zuiderent, S. "A Feeling for Data—Screening and Researching Prostate Cancer with Care." In *Prostatan—det ständiga gisslet? Mannen och prostatan I kultur, medicin och historia*, edited by M. Björkman. Lund: Nordic Academic Press, 2018.

Johannison, K. *Den mörka kontinenten*. Stockholm: Norstedts, 1994.

Johnson, E. *Gendering Drugs: Feminist Studies of Pharmaceuticals*. London: Palgrave Macmillan, 2017.

Johnson, E. *Refracting through Technologies: Bodies, Medical Technologies and Norms*. London: Routledge, 2019.

Johnson, E., E. Sjögren, and C. Åsberg. *Glocal Pharma: International Brands and the Imagination of Local Masculinity*. London: Routledge, 2016.

Jordanova, L. *Nature Displayed: Gender, Science and Medicine 1760–1820*. London: Longman, 1999.

Jülich, S. "The Making of a Best-Selling Book on Reproduction: Lennart Nilsson's *A Child Is Born*." *Bulletin of the History of Medicine*, 89, no. 3 (2015): 491–525.

Juth, N., and C. Munthe. *The Ethics of Screening in Health Care and Medicine*. Heidelberg: Springer Verlag, 2012.

Kalager, M., M. Zelen, F. Langmark, and H-O. Adami. "Effect of Screening Mammography on Breast-Cancer Mortality in Norway." *New England Journal of Medicine* 363, no. 13 (2010): 1203–1210.

Kellogg Parsons, J. "Modifiable Risk Factors for Benign Prostatic Hyperplasia and Lower Urinary Tract Symptoms: New Approaches to Old Problems." *Journal of Urology* 178, no. 2 (2007): 395–401.

Kenny, K., A. Broom, E. Kirby, J. Oliffe, D. Wyld, and Z. Lwin. "Reciprocity, Autonomy, and Vulnerability in Men's Experiences of Informal Cancer Care." *Qualitative Health Research* 30, no. 4 (2019): 491–503.

King, S. *Pink Ribbons, Inc.: Breast Cancer and the Politics of Philanthropy*. Minneapolis: University of Minnesota Press, 2006.

Kinn, A-C., et al. *Prostata—mannens ständiga gissel*. Södertälje: Astra Sverige, 1997.

Kirmayer, L. J. "Culture and the Metaphoric Mediation of Pain." *Transcultural Psychiatry* 45, no. 2 (2008): 318–338.

Klawiter, M. *The Biopolitics of Breast Cancer: Changing Cultures of Disease and Activism*. Minneapolis: University of Minnesota Press, 2008.

Kleinman, A. "Depression, Somatization and the 'New Cross-Cultural Psychiatry'." *Social Science and Medicine* 11, no. 1 (1977): 3–10.

Klestinec, C. "A History of Anatomy Theaters in Sixteenth-Century Padua." *Journal of the History of Medicine and Allied Sciences* 59, no. 3 (2004): 375–412.

Kopytoff, I. "The Cultural Biography of Things: Commoditization as Process." In *The Social Life of Things: Commodities in Cultural Perspective*, edited by A. Appadurai, 64–91. New York: Cambridge University Press, 1986.

Kretschmer, H. L. "Electrosection of the Prostate." Chicago: Presbyterian Hospital (Undated, offprint), 1932[?].

Kretschmer, H. L. "Prostatic Obstruction from the Life Insurance Point of View." New York: Association of Life Insurance Medical Directors of America, 1936.

Krieger, J., L. Nyberg, and J. Nickel. "NIH Consensus Definition and Classification of Prostatitis." *Journal of the American Medical Association* 282, no. 3 (1999): 236–237.

Kruse, C. "The Bayesian Approach to Forensic Evidence: Evaluating, Communicating, and Distributing Responsibility." *Social Studies of Science* 43, no. 5 (2012): 657–680.

Latour, B. "On the Partial Existence of Existing and Non-Existing Objects." In *Biographies of Scientific Objects*, edited by L. Daston, 247–269. Chicago: University of Chicago Press, 2000.

Latour, B. *Science in Action: How to Follow Scientists and Engineers through Society*. Cambridge, MA: Harvard University Press, 1987.

Latour, B., and S. Woolgar. *Laboratory Life: The Construction of Scientific Facts*. New York: Sage Publications, 1979.

Leder, D. *The Absent Body*. Chicago: University of Chicago Press, 1990.

Lee, T. K., A. B. Handy, W. Kwan, J. L. Oliffe, L. A. Brotto, R. J. Wassersug, and G. W. Dowsett. "The Impact of Prostate Cancer Treatment on the Sexual Quality of Life for Men-Who-Have-Sex-With-Men." *Journal of Sexual Medicine* 12, no. 12 (2015): 2378–2386.

Leigh, D. A. (1993) "Prostatitis—An Increasing Clinical Problem for Diagnosis and Management." *Journal of Antimicrobial Chemotherapy* 32, suppl. A (1993): 1–9.

Lindén, L. "Moving Evidence: Patient Groups, Biomedicine and Affects." *Science, Technology and Human Values* 35, no. 4 (2020): 444–473.

Loe, M. *The Rise of Viagra: How the Little Blue Pill Changed Sex in America*. New York: New York University Press, 2004.

Lundström, C. "White Ethnography: (Un)comfortable Conveniences and Shared Privileges in Field Work with Swedish Migrant Women." *NORA—Nordic Journal of Feminist and Gender Research* 18, no. 2 (2010): 70–87.

Lupton, D. *The Quantified Self: A Sociology of Self-Tracking*. Cambridge: Polity Press, 2016.

Macefield, R. C., J. A. Lane, C. Metcalfe, L. Down, et al. "Do the Risk Factors of Age, Family History of Prostate Cancer or a Higher Prostate Specific Antigen Level Raise Anxiety at Prostate Biopsy?" *European Journal of Cancer* 45, no. 14 (2009): 2569–2573.

Maldonado, O. "Price-Effectiveness: Pharmacoeconomics, Value and the Right Price for HPV Vaccines." *Journal of Cultural Economy* 10, no. 2 (2017): 163–177.

Maldonado Castañeda, O. "Ett hälsosamt tillstånd av ovisshet. Tankar kring PSA-prov, förutsägbarhet och sårbarhet." In *Prostatan— det ständiga gisslet? Mannen och prostatan I kultur, medicin och historia*, edited by M. Björkman, 59–73. Lund: Nordic Academic Press, 2018.

Maron, P. "Living Well with a Healthy Weight: A Case of the Body Mass Index as a Governing Practice." In manuscript.

Marshall, B. "'Hard Science': Gender Constructions of Sexual Dysfunction in the 'Viagra Age'." *Sexualities* 5, no. 2 (2002): 131–158.

Marshall, B. "The New Virility: Viagra, Male Aging and Sexual Function." *Sexualities* 9, no. 3 (2006): 345–362.

Martin, E. "The Egg and the Sperm: How Science Has Constructed a Romance Based on Stereotypical Male-Female Roles." *Signs* 16, no. 3 (1991): 485–501.

Martin, E. *The Woman in the Body: A Cultural Analysis of Reproduction.* Boston: Beacon Press, 1987.

Martin, S. C., Jr., ed. *Prostatic Hypertrophy from Every Surgical Standpoint by George M. Phillips, M.D. and Forty Distinguished Authorities.* St. Louis: AJOD Company, Medical Publishers, 1903.

Marx, F. J., and A. Karenberg. "History of the Term Prostate." *The Prostate* 69 (2009): 208–213.

Marx, F. J., and A. Karenberg. "Uro-Words Making History: Ureter and Urethra." *The Prostate* 70 (2010): 952–958.

McCracken, L., and C. Eccleston. "Coping or Acceptance: What to Do about Chronic Pain?" *Pain* 105, nos. 1–2 (2003): 197–204.

McLaren, A. *Impotence: A Cultural History.* Chicago: University of Chicago Press, 2007.

Meyer, M., and J. Dykes. "Criteria for Rigor in Visualization Design Study." *IEEE Transactions on Visualization and Computer Graphics* 26, no. 1 (2020): 87–97.

Miksad, R., G. Bubley, P. Church, et al. "Prostate Cancer in a Transgender Woman 41 Years after Initiation of Feminization." *Journal of the American Medical Association* 296, no. 19 (2006): 2312–2317.

Mol, A. M. *The Body Multiple: Ontology in Medical Practice.* Durham: Duke University Press, 2002.

Moscucci, O. *The Science of Woman: Gynaecology and Gender in England, 1800–1929.* Cambridge: Cambridge University Press, 1993.

Moser, I. "A Body That Matters? The Role of Embodiment in the Recomposition of Life after a Road Traffic Accident." *Scandinavian Journal of Disability Research* 11, no. 2 (2009): 83–99.

Murphy, M. *Seizing the Means of Reproduction: Entanglements of Feminism, Health and Technoscience.* Durham, NC: Duke University Press, 2012.

Mustafa N., G. Einstein, M. MacNeill, and J. Watt-Watson. "The Lived Experiences of Chronic Pain among Immigrant Indian-Canadian Women: A Phenomenological Analysis." *Canadian Journal of Pain* 4, no. 3 (2020): 40–50.

National Cancer Centre Singapore. "Prostate Cancer." https://www.nccs.com.sg/PatientCare/WhatisCancer/TypesofCancer/Pages/Prostate-Cancer.aspx, accessed September 2020.

O'Leary, M. "Validity of the 'Bother Score' in the Evaluation and Treatment of Symptomatic Benign Prostatic Hyperplasia." *Review of Urology* 7, no. 1 (2005): 1–10.

Oliffe, J. L. "Embodied Masculinity and Androgen Deprivation Therapy." *Sociology of Health and Illness* 28, no. 4 (2006): 410–432.

Oliffe, J. L., M. Halpin, J. L. Bottorff, T. G. Hislop, M. McKenzie, and L. Mroz. "How Prostate Cancer Support Groups Do and Do Not Survive: British Columbian Perspectives." *American Journal of Men's Health* 2, no. 2 (2008): 143–155.

O'Shea, C. D. "'A Plea for the Prostate': Doctors, Prostate Dysfunction, and Male Sexuality in Late 19th- and Early 20th-Century Canada." *Canadian Bulletin of Medical History* 29, no. 1 (2012): 7–27.

Oudshoorn, N. *Beyond the Natural Body.* London: Routledge, 1994.

Oudshoorn, N. *The Male Pill.* Durham: Duke University Press, 2003.

Overall, G. W. *A Synopsis of Reprints on the treatment of Stricture, Urethritis, Prostatitis, Cystitis, Impotency and Spermatorrhea with Electricity, Cataphoresis and allied remedies, as taken from the Mississippi Valley*

Medical Journal of—, 1883, and August, 1887; Medical Mirror of April, 1896, and the Journal of the American Medical Association of January 21st, 1899, etc. HNM Semmelweis Medical History Library, Budapest (unknown publisher and publishing year; estimated publishing year is 1900 as the latest mentioned print is 1899), 23–25.

Parks, T. *Teach Us to Sit Still: A Sceptic's Search for Health and Healing.* London: Harvill Secker, 2001.

Parsons, T. *Social Structure and Dynamic Process: The Case of Modern Medical Practice.* London: Routledge, 1951.

Penner, B. *Bathroom.* London: Reaktion Books, Objekt Series, 2014.

Perletti, G., E. Marras, F. M. E. Wagenlehner, and V. Magri. "Antimicrobial Therapy for Chronic Bacterial Prostatitis." *Cochrane Database of Systematic Reviews* 8, no. CD009071 (2013).

Perlman, G. "Looking Back: Engaging Prostate Cancer as a Gay Man." In *Gay and Bisexual Men Living with Prostate Cancer from Diagnosis to Recovery,* edited by J. M. Ussher, J. Perz, and B. R. S. Rosser, 297–303. New York: Harrington Park Press.

Perlman, G. *What Every Gay Man Needs to Know about Prostate Cancer.* New York: Magnus Books, 2013.

Perović, M., D. Jacobson, E. Glazer, C. Pukall, and G. Einstein. "Are You in Pain If You Say You Are Not? Accounts of Pain in Somali-Canadian Women with Female Genital Cutting (FGC)." *Pain* 162, no. 4 (2020): 1144–1152.

Persson, A. "An Unintended Side Effect of Pepper Spray: Gender Trouble and 'Repair Work' in an Armed Forces Unit." *Men and Masculinities* 15, no. 2 (2012): 132–151.

Peters, T., J. Donovan, H. Kay, P. Abrams, J. de la Rosette, D. Porru, J. Ghüroff, et al. "The International Continence Society 'Benign Prostatic Hyperplasia' Study: The Bothersomeness of Urinary Symptoms." *Journal of Urology* 157 (1997): 885–889.

Polkey, J. "Incomplete Late Results after Supra-Pubic Prostatectomy." *Urologic and Cutaneous Review* 30 (1926): 65–74.

Porter, T. "Life Insurance, Medical Testing, and the Management of Mortality." In *Biographies of Scientific Objects*, edited by L. Daston, 226–246. Chicago: University of Chicago Press, 2000.

Potts, A. "Deleuze on Viagra (or, What can a 'Viagra-Body' Do?)." *Body and Society* 10, no. 1 (2004): 17–36.

Rice, S. M., J. S. Oliffe, M. T. Kelly, P. Cormie, S. Chambers, J. S. Ogrodniczuk, and D. Kealy. "Depression and Prostate Cancer: Examining Comorbidity and Male-Specific Symptoms." *American Journal of Men's Health* 12, no. 6 (2018): 1864–1872.

Robertson, S. *Understanding Men and Health: Masculinities, Identity and Well-Being*. Maidenhead, UK: Open University Press, 2007.

Rodriguez, S. *Female Circumcision and Clitoridectomy in the United States: A History of a Medical Treatment*. Rochester, NY: Boydell & Brewer, 2018.

Rosenfeld, D., and C. Faircloth, eds., *Medicalized Masculinities*. Philadelphia: Temple University Press, 2006.

Rosser, B. R. S., S. Hunt, B. Capistrant, N. Kohli, B. Konety, D. Mitteldorf, M. Ross, K. Talley, and W. West. "Understanding Prostate Cancer in Gay, Bisexual, and Other Men Who Have Sex with Men and Transgender Women." In *Gay and Bisexual Men Living with Prostate Cancer from Diagnosis to Recovery*, edited by J. M. Ussher, J. Perz, and B. R. S. Rosser, 12–37. New York: Harrington Park Press, 2018.

Sagen, E., *Transurethral Resection of the Prostate. Studies on Efficacy, Morbidity and Costs*. Academic dissertation, University of Gothenburg, 2020

Sakharkar, P., and A. Kahaleh. "Age and Racial/Ethnic Disparities and Burden of Prostate Cancer: A Cross Sectional Population Based Study." *Journal of Basic and Clinical Pharmacy* 8 (2017): S022–S026.

Sandberg, L. "Closer to Touch: Sexuality, Embodiment and Masculinity in Older Men's Lives." In *Ageing in Everyday Life: Materialities and Embodiments*, edited by S. Katz, 129–144. Bristol, UK: Policy Press, 2018.

Sarma, A., D. Jacobson, M. McGree, R. Roberts, M. Lieber, and S. Jacobsen. "A Population Based Study of Incidence and Treatment of Benign Prostatic Hyperplasia Among Residents of Olmsted County, Minnesota: 1987–1997." *Journal of Urology* 173 (2005): 2048–2053.

Scarry, E. *The Body in Pain*. Oxford: Oxford University Press, 1988.

Schiebinger, L. *Nature's Body: Gender in the Making of Modern Science*. Boston: Beacon Press, 1993.

Schillmeier, M. *Rethinking Disability. Bodies, Senses and Things*. London: Routledge, 2010.

Schlomm, T. "The Era of Prostate-Specific Antigen-Based Personalized Prostate Cancer Screening Has Only Just Begun." *European Urology* 68, no. 2 (2015): 2014–2015.

Schröder, F. H., J. Hugosson, M. J. Roobol, L. J. Teuvo, et al. "Screening and Prostate-Cancer Mortality in a Randomized European Study." *New England Journal of Medicine* 360 (2009): 1320–1328.

Sengoopta, C. *The Most Secret Quintessence of Life: Sex, Glands, and Hormones, 1850–1950*. Chicago: University of Chicago Press, 2006.

Shackley, D. "A Century of Prostatic Surgery." *BJU International* 83, no. 7 (1999): 776–782.

Shotwell, R. "Animals, Pictures, and Skeletons: Andreas Vesalius's Reinvention of the Public Anatomy Lesson." *Journal of the History of Medicine and Allied Sciences* 71, no. 1 (2015): 1–18.

Socialstyrelsen. "Mer forskning om prostatacancerscreening behövs." https://www.socialstyrelsen.se/om-socialstyrelsen/pressrum/press/mer -forskning-om-prostatacancerscreening-behovs/, 12 February 2018.

Socialstyrelsen. "Om PSA-prov—för att hunna upptäcka prostatacancer i ett tidigt skede—fördelar och nackdelar." Art. no. 2014-8-4 (4 August 2014): 1–6. https://www.socialstyrelsen.se/globalassets/share point-dokument/artikelkatalog/kunskapsstod/2014-8-4.pdf

Socialstyrelsen. "Prostatacancer, screening med PSA-prov kompletterat med annat diagnostikt test." https://www.socialstyrelsen.se

/regler-och-riktlinjer/nationella-screeningprogram/slutliga-rekom mendationer/prostatacancer/, 2018.

Solnit, R. "Drawing the Constellation." In *Meridel Rubenstein: Belonging. Los Alamos to Vietnam, Photoworks and Installations*, by J. Crump, L. R. Lippard, E. Scarry, R. Solnit, and T. Tempest William, 72–75. Los Angeles: St. Ann's Press, 2004.

Solnit, R. *Storming the Gates of Paradise: Landscapes for Politics*. Oakland: University of California Press, 2007.

Sontag, S. *Illness as Metaphor*. New York: Farrar, Straus & Giroux, 1978.

Statens Beredning för Medicinsk och Social Utvärdering (SBU). *Godartad prostataförstoring med avflödeshinder. En systematisk litteraturöversikt*. Swedish Council on Health Technology Assessment, 2011.

Steinberg, P. *A Salamander's Tale*. New York: Skyhorse, 2015.

STHLM3 [Stockholm3 test]. "About STHLM3." www.sthlm3.se, accessed September 2020.

Stone, N., and E. Crawford. "To Screen or Not to Screen: The Prostate Cancer Dilemma." *Asian Journal of Andrology* 17, no. 1 (2015): 44–45.

Straits Times. "Prostate Cancer Screening Better with New Thinking." https://www.straitstimes.com/singapore/health/prostate-cancer -screening-better-with-new-thinking, 5 October 2016.

Suchman, L. *Human-Machine Reconfigurations: Plans and Situated Actions*. 2nd ed. Cambridge: Cambridge University Press, 2007.

SVD Svenska Dagbladet. "Skånska män erbjuds Prostataprov." https:// www.svd.se/man-i-skane-erbjuds-prostataprov *Svenska Dagbladet*, 26 June 2018.

Swift, A. "Understanding Pain and the Human Body's Response to It." *Nursing Times* 114, no. 3 (2018): 22–26.

Tangpricha, V., and M. den Heijer. "Oestrogen and Anti-Androgen Therapy for Transgender Women." *The Lancet—Diabetes and Endocrinology* 5, no. 4 (2017): 291–300.

Thaxton, L., J. G. Emshoff, and O. Guessous. "Prostate Cancer Support Groups." *Journal of Psychosocial Oncology* 23, no. 1 (2005): 25–40.

Thompson, C. *Making Parents. The Ontological Choreography of Reproductive Technologies*. Cambridge, MA: MIT Press, 2005.

Thompson, H. *The Diseases of the Prostate: Their Pathology and Treatment*. London: J. & A. Churchill, 1873.

Thorsén, D. "Epidemins aktörer. Patientkollektiv som maktfaktor: exemplet hiv/aids." *Socialmedicinsk tidskrift* 92, no. 6 (2016): 717–715.

Thum, S., B. Haben, G. Christ, and R. Sen Gupta. "[Female prostate cancer?]" *Pathologe* 38, no. 5 (2017): 448–450.

Tiefer, L. "The Viagra Phenomenon." *Sexualities* 9, no. 3 (2006): 273–294.

Timmermans, S., and M. Buchbinder. "Newborn Screening and Maternal Diagnosis: Rethinking Family Benefit." *Social Science and Medicine* 73, no. 7 (2011): 1014–1018.

Timmermans, S., and B. Marc. *The Gold Standard: The Challenge of Evidence-Based Medicine and Standardization in Healthcare*. Philadelphia: Temple University Press, 2003.

Tuana, N. "The Speculum of Ignorance: The Women's Health Movement and Epistemologies of Ignorance." *Hypatia* 21, no. 3 (2006): 1–19.

Turo, R., S. Jallad, S. Prescott, and W. Cross. "Metastatic Prostate Cancer in Transsexual Diagnosed after Three Decades of Estrogen Therapy." *Canadian Urology Association* 7, nos. 7–8 (2013): E544–E546.

UK NSC (National Screening Committee). "UK NSC Prostate Cancer Screening Recommendation." September 2014.

UK NSC (National Screening Committee). "The UK NSC Recommendation on Prostate Cancer Screening/PSA Testing in Men over the Age of 50." https://legacyscreening.phe.org.uk/prostatecancer, January 2016.

Underman, K. *Feeling Medicine: How the Pelvic Exam Shapes Medical Training*. New York: New York University Press, 2020.

Unsigned. "Hypertrophy of the Prostate and Gay Attire." *Urologic and Cutaneous Review* 28 (1924): 251–253.

Ussher, J. M., J. Perz, and B. R. S. Rosser, eds. *Gay and Bisexual Men Living with Prostate Cancer from Diagnosis to Recovery*. New York: Harrington Park Press, 2018.

Uustal, E. "Debatt: Nya strategier för behandling av långvarig bäckensmärta." *Läkartidningen*. https://lakartidningen.se/Opinion/Debatt /2016/12/Nya-strategier-for-behandling-av-langvarig-backensmarta/, accessed September 2020.

Valier, H. K. "The Problematic Prehistory of Prostate Cancer" and "Screening, Patients, and the Politics of Prevention." In *A History of Prostate Cancer: Cancer, Men and Medicine*, chs. 2 and 6. London: Palgrave Macmillan, 2016.

Vander Veer, J. *Clinical Aspect of the Enlarged Prostate, with a Review of 67 Cases*. Reprinted from the *New York State Journal of Medicine* 1909 and read at 3rd District Branch of the Medical Society of the State of New York, Troy, October 27, 1908.

Van Dijck, J. *The Transparent Body: A Cultural Analysis of Medical Imaging*. Seattle: University of Washington Press, 2015.

Viney, W., F. Callard, and A. Woods. "Critical Medical Humanities: Embracing Entanglement, Taking Risks." *Medical Humanities* 41 (2015): 2–7.

Vogel, E. "Restoring the Balance: Living Well with Pain." *Somatosphere: Science, Medicine and Anthropology*. http://somatosphere.net/2019 /restoring-the-balance-living-well-with-pain.html/, 16 April 2019.

Wailoo, K. *Drawing Blood: Technology and Disease Identity in Twentieth-Century America*. Baltimore: Johns Hopkins University Press, 1997.

Wailoo, K. *How Cancer Crossed the Color Line*. Oxford: Oxford University Press, 2011.

Wailoo, K., J. Livingston, S. Epstein, and R. Aronowitz. *Three Shots at Prevention: The HPV Vaccine and the Politics of Medicine's Simple Solutions*. Baltimore: Johns Hopkins University Press, 2010.

Waldby, C. *The Visible Human Project: Informatic Bodies and Posthuman Medicine*. London: Routledge, 2000.

Walton, G. "Hysteria, as Affected by Removal of the Ovaries." *Boston Medical and Surgical Journal* 110, no. 23 (1884): 529.

Wassersug, R. "Getting Your PSA Checked Is Good for Overall Health." *Trends in Urology and Men's Health* (March/April 2016): 15–16.

Whitehead, A., and A. Woods, eds., *The Edinburgh Companion to the Critical Medical Humanities*. Edinburgh: Edinburgh University Press, 2016.

Williams, J. S., P. Martin, and J. Gabe. "The Pharmaceuticalisation of Society? A Framework for Analysis." *Sociology of Health and Illness* 33, no. 5 (2011): 710–725.

Wilson, J. M. G., and J. Jungner. "Principles and Practice of Screening for Disease." Public Health Paper 34. Geneva: World Health Organization, 1968.

Winterich, J., S. Quandt, J. Grzywacz, P. Clark, D. Miller, J. Acuna, and T. Arcury. "Masculinity and the Body: How African American and White Men Experience Cancer Screening Exams Involving the Rectum." *American Journal of Men's Health* 3, no. 4 (2009): 300–309.

Wright, M., A. Wren, T. Somer, M. Goetz, A. Fras, B. Huh, L. Rogers, and F. Keefe. "Pain Acceptance, Hope, and Optimism: Relationships to Pain Adjustment in Patients with Chronic Musculoskeletal Pain." *Journal of Pain* 12, no. 11 (2011): 1155–1162.

Young, H. *Studies on Hypertrophy and Cancer of the Prostate*. Johns Hopkins Hospital Reports Vol. XIV. Baltimore: Johns Hopkins University Press, 1906.

Zeiler, K. "An Analytic Framework for Conceptualizations of Disease: Nine Structuring Questions and How Some Conceptualizations of

Alzheimer's Disease Can Lead to Diseasisation." *Medicine, Health Care and Philosophy* 23, no. 4 (2020): 677–693.

Zeiler, K. "A Phenomenological Analysis of Bodily Self-Awareness in the Experience of Pain and Pleasure: On Dys-Appearance and Eu-Appearance." *Medical Health Care and Philosophy* 13, no. 4 (2010): 333–342.

Zeiler, K., and L. Guntram. "Sexed Embodiment in Atypical Pubertal Development: Intersubjectivity, Excorporation, and the Importance of Making Space for Difference." In *Feminist Phenomenology and Medicine*, edited by L. F. Käll and K. Zeiler, 141–160. Albany, NY: SUNY Press, 2014.

Zeiler, K., and L. Käll. "Still Alice? Ethical Aspects of Conceptualising Selfhood in Dementia." In *The Routledge Handbook of the Medical Humanities*, edited by A. Bleakley, 290–299. London: Routledge, 2020.

Zuiderent-Jerak, T. *Situated Intervention: Sociological Experiments in Health Care*. Cambridge, MA: MIT Press, 2015.

Index